DIAGNOSTIC PICTURE TESTS IN

CLINICAL SURGERY

William F. Walker

DSc, ChM, FRCS, FRCS (Ed), FRSE
Emeritus Professor of Surgery
Ninewells Hospital, Dundee
Dundee University

GW00675821

Wolfe Publishing Ltd

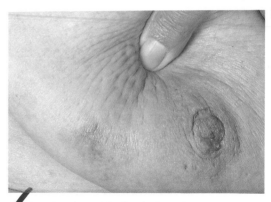

1 (a) What does this sign indicate?
(b) What causes the pitting?
(c) What investigations should be carried out?
(d) What treatments may be given?
(e) Is there a different regime in the elderly, i.e. over 70 years of age?
(f) What new idea has been suggested in mastectomy?

2 (a) What is this lesion and what is its likely cause?
(b) What treatment is required?
(c) What secondary condition may be involved?
(d) What future treatment may be required?

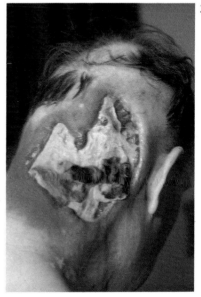

3

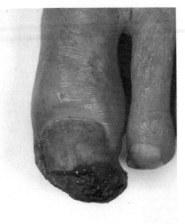

3 (a) What is present in this big toe?
(b) Why was there bleeding?
(c) What procedure is necessary and what is the diagnosis?
(d) What operation should be done?
(e) What are the commonest sites of this condition?
(f) What is the most important determinant of malignancy?
(g) What therapies may be helpful?

4

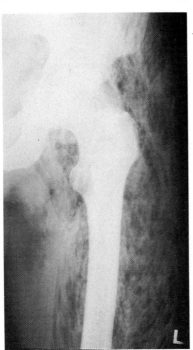

4 (a) What is shown in this plain X-ray?
(b) What are the causes?
(c) What organisms are involved?
(d) What treatment is helpful?

5 (a) What has this baby developed?
(b) How may this have occurred?
(c) What investigations should be done?
(d) What dangers may arise from the condition?
(e) What treatment cleared up the problem?

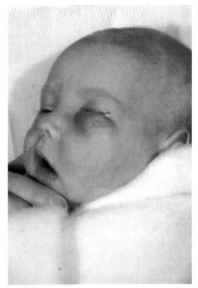

6 (a) What are the distinguishing features of this disease?
(b) What conditions may cause it?
(c) How is the diagnosis established?
(d) What treatment can be given?
(e) What operation may be necessary?

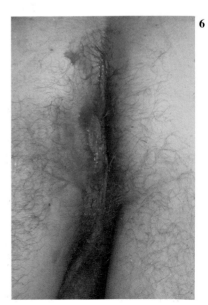

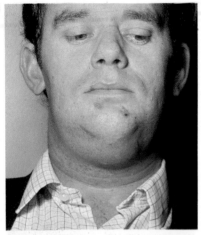

7 (a) What is this inflammatory swelling called?
(b) At what level is the inflammatory process?
(c) What problem may arise from the swelling?
(d) What organisms are involved?
(e) If incision is required, what dangers may arise?

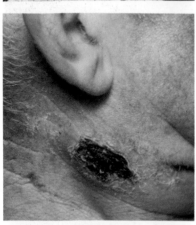

8 (a) What does this black ulcer suggest?
(b) Does it help to know that he is a farmer?
(c) How does this condition occur?
(d) On examination what would be looked for?
(e) How is the diagnosis confirmed?

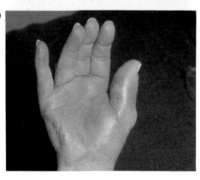

9 (a) What is seen in this man's hand?
(b) How may this have started?
(c) What further consequences may arise?
(d) How would these be dealt with?
(e) What may result from this infection and any subsequent surgery?

10 (a) This lesion developed in a few weeks and later an ulcer appeared. What does this suggest?

(b) What might be another diagnosis had the progress been slower?

(c) What are the usual characteristics of the lesion shown?

(d) How is it treated?

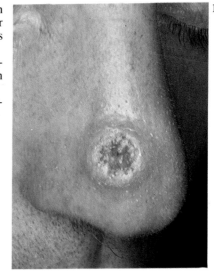

11 This patient was admitted with a gross swelling of his face and enlarged glands in his neck, especially on the right side.

(a) What clinical assessment could be made?

(b) Would the nature of his work give an idea as to his disease?

(c) How would his work be a cause of his problem?

(d) What is the diagnosis?

(e) What other types of this disease are possible?

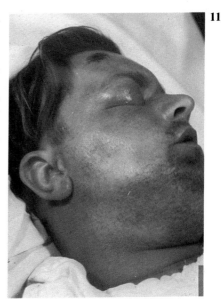

12 (a) What is the lesion shown?
(b) How has it occurred?
(c) What name is given to it?
(d) How should it be dealt with?

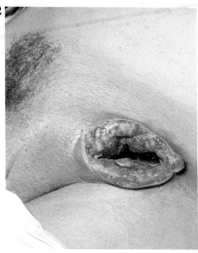

13 (a) What does the visible redness behind the knee suggest?
(b) What would you expect to feel?
(c) What investigation would be helpful?
(d) How should the condition be dealt with?

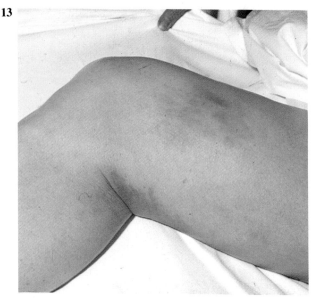

14 (a) What operation is being carried out?
(b) What are the symptoms of the condition?
(c) What other conditions may mimic this condition?
(d) What investigations should be done prior to surgery?
(e) What are the requisites for surgery?

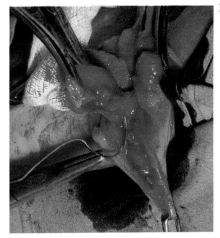

15 This patient had a swelling since birth. Various attempts were made to improve it.
(a) What is the lesion likely to be?
(b) What signs would support this?
(c) What special investigation should be done?
(d) How may it be more possible now to deal with this problem?
(e) What is Branham's sign?

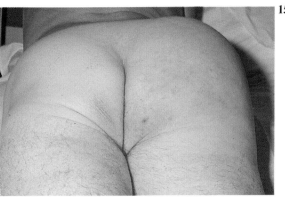

16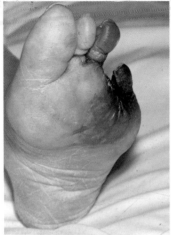

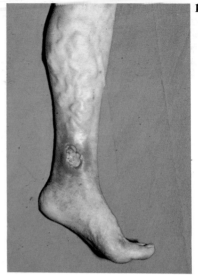 **17**

16 An *ischaemic foot* is present with dry and moist gangrene.
(a) What is the main cause of the problem?
(b) What investigations should be done?
(c) What operation was done?
(d) How could blood flow be investigated?
(e) Could the foot be saved?

17 (a) What type of ulcer is present?
(b) What are the characteristics of this type of ulcer?
(c) What is the effect on the large veins?
(d) What other factors related to chronic ulcers may delay healing?

18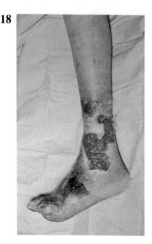

18 (a) What type of ulcer is shown and what is it caused by?
(b) What are the characteristics of such ulcer?
(c) What is usually present to indicate the type of ulcer?
(d) Are these ulcers related to varicose veins?

19 (a) What does this girl's facies suggest?
(b) What condition causes this?
(c) What are the early symptoms?
(d) How is the condition often transmitted?
(e) What treatment is required?

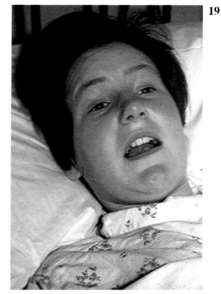

20 (a) What is the diagnosis of the lesion in this man's lower lip?
(b) What operation should be done?
(c) Would radiotherapy be required?
(d) How successful would the operation be?

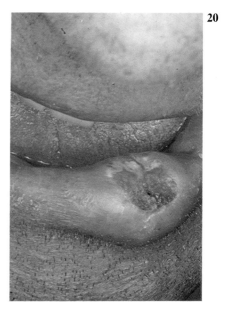

21 (a) What is visible on the tongue?

(b) What are the possible causes?

(c) What investigations should be done?

(d) There is culture positive for a *tubercle*: where else in the tongue should you look for an ulcer?

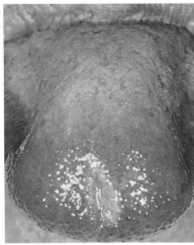

22 (a) A swelling is obvious on the right side of the tongue. What are the possibilities?

(b) How is the diagnosis made?

(c) What tumours may be present in the tongue?

(d) What is the commonest tumour of the tongue?

(e) How are malignant tumours classified?

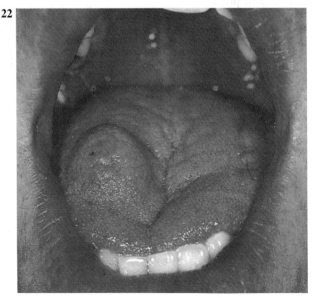

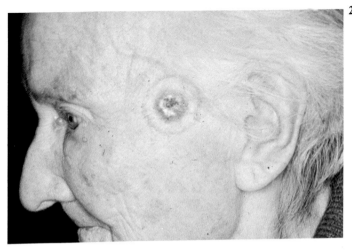

23 (a) A typical example of this lesion. What is it?
  (b) What are the characteristics?
  (c) Are the lymph glands involved?
  (d) What treatments might be of value?

24 (a) Why have we photographed this woman from above?
  (b) What symptoms may be present?
  (c) What sign may become manifest?
  (d) What investigations would help in diagnosis?
  (e) How should the condition be treated?

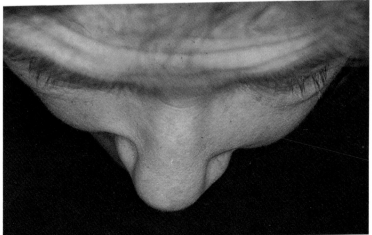

25

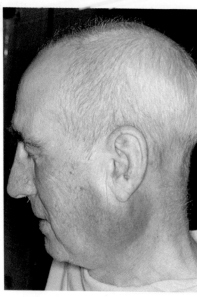

25 (a) What is the cause of the swelling on the left side of the face?
(b) What observation would support the presence of an abscess?
(c) Why is this condition so painful?
(d) How common is this condition?
(e) What type of patients get it?
(f) How is it dealt with?

26

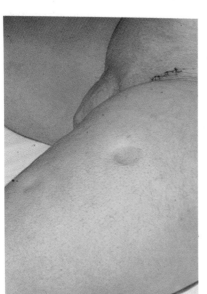

26 (a) What is shown here?
(b) What types are these?
(c) What is the cause of the primary condition?
(d) What is the cause of the secondary condition?

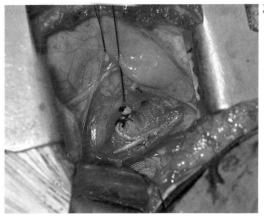

27 (a) The chest has been opened on the left side. What is demonstrated?
(b) How is the lesion detected clinically?
(c) How is the diagnosis made?
(d) What nerve may be in danger during the operation?

28 (a) A section of the aorta is shown. What is present?
(b) How is it detected?
(c) What can result from the lesion?
(d) What is required to be done?

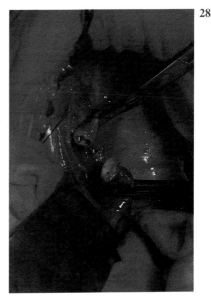

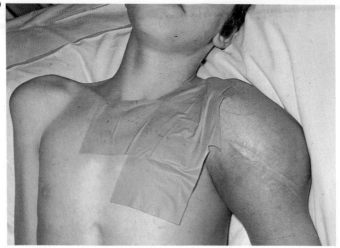

29 (a) A 15-year-old boy developed a swelling in his left humerus. What is the likely diagnosis?
(b) What sex does this occur in predominantly and at what likely age?
(c) Does the lesion spread?
(d) What therapy could be used?
(e) Does the condition occur over the age of 20 years?

30

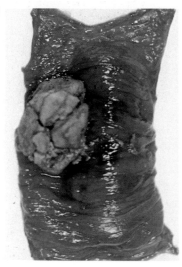

30 (a) What is the name given to this problem?
(b) How does the problem arise?
(c) How is the obstruction produced?
(d) Can it come from a nucleus of a gallstone?
(e) How is the condition managed?

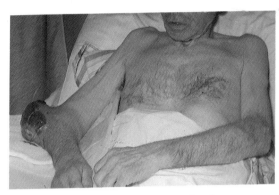

31 (a) What is the lesion in this patient?
(b) Is it a primary or a secondary tumour?
(c) What is the most likely primary site?
(d) How would it be treated?
(e) What is the result likely to be?

32 (a) This tumour developed from the sacrococcygeal region. What is it?
(b) What type of tumour is it?
(c) Where do these appear?
(d) How should it be treated?

33 (a) This slow growing tumour in a middle-aged man is not common. What might it be?
(b) What is its origin?
(c) Where, therefore, are the common sites?
(d) What is the rate of progress?
(e) Can surgery help?

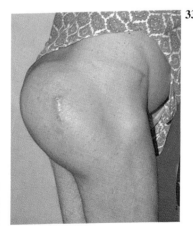

34

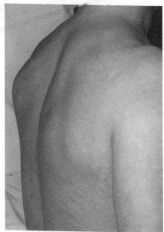

34 (a) This patient presented with a firm swelling on the back of his shoulder. What is the likely diagnosis?
(b) How is the diagnosis confirmed?
(c) What type of tumour is it?
(d) Where do they usually occur?
(e) What is the survival period?

35 (a) What is the likely diagnosis of this rapidly growing, hard, fixed tumour?
(b) What is its histological type?
(c) What treatment should be given?
(d) What is the prognosis?

36 (a) What might be the diagnosis of this fairly rapidly growing tumour of the buttock?
(b) What are the types of this tumour?
(c) What differentiates between the types?
(d) What are the differences in treatment between the types?

35

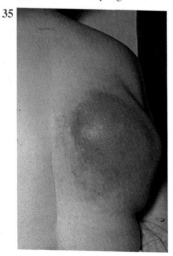

36

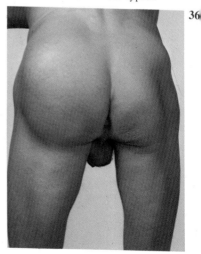

37 (a) This patient complained of sudden severe abdominal pain. What is the problem?
(b) How does this occur?
(c) What can result from this?
(d) Is it a common condition?
(e) What operation should be carried out?

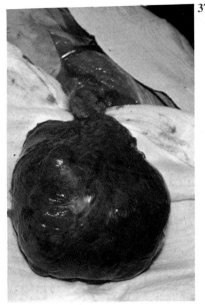

38 (a) What problem is shown in the X-ray?
(b) What signs and symptoms would be present?
(c) What are the causes that produce the problems?
(d) How is the diagnosis supported?
(e) What treatment would be advised?

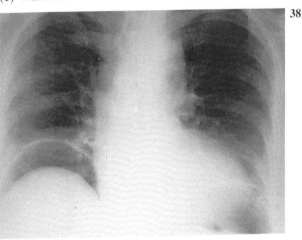

39

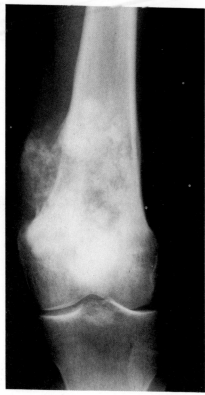

39 (a) What is the diagnosis and at what age is this usually seen?
(b) What are the clinical features?
(c) What does the X-ray show?
(d) Where are the metastases found?
(e) What treatment could be used?

40 (a) The specimen shows what characteristic of an intestinal resection?
(b) What is the 'appendage'?
(c) What symptoms would alert you to the diagnosis?
(d) What investigations could be done?

40

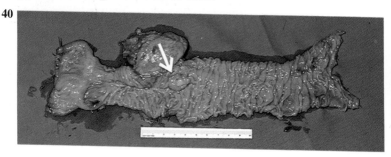

41 (a) What fluid is draining out from the opening in the abdomen?

(b) How could this have happened?

(c) The drainage continued for months, how was it stopped?

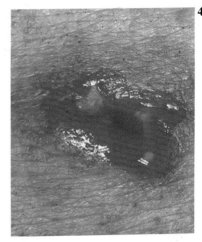

42 (a) This pathological specimen illustrates a number of problems, what are they?

(b) What type of tumour is in the ureter?

(c) What is the first sign of its presence?

(d) What investigations should be made?

(e) What area of the ureter is the most difficult to diagnose as carcinomatous?

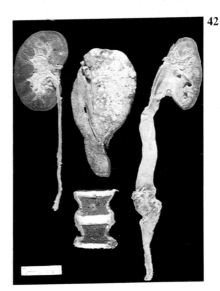

43

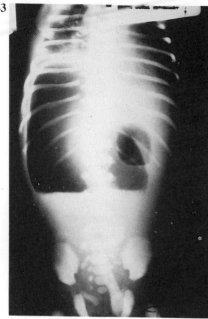

43 (a) What does this X-ray show?
(b) What is the cause of the problem?
(c) What is the sex ratio?
(d) What are the clinical features of the condition?
(e) What treatment is required?

44

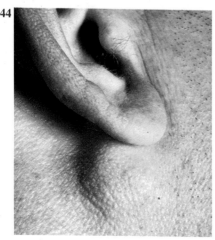

44 This patient presented with a swelling below the lobe of the ear.
(a) What is the most likely cause?
(b) What are the characteristics?
(c) What is the name given to the condition?
(d) What other diagnoses are possible?
(e) Histologically, what is the lesion made of?

45 (a) The swelling in this patient is very near the ear lobe. What are the possibilities?
(b) What would support it being a mixed parotid tumour?
(c) What is the histology?
(d) Is it totally benign?

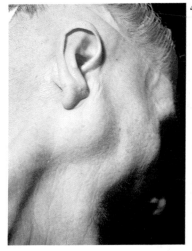

46 (a) What is visible in this patient's mouth?
(b) What investigations are required?
(c) Sialogram showed a large stone in the duct adjacent to the gland. What should be done?
(d) What are the dangers of operation?

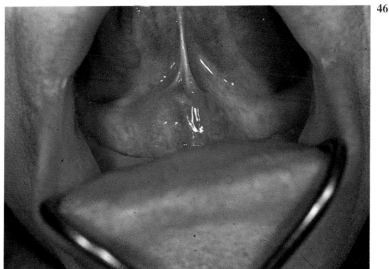

47

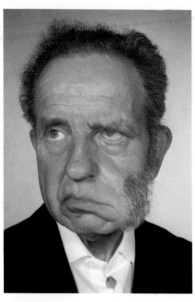

47 (a) What would you deduce from the facial expression of this man?

(b) What other problems may this cause?

(c) Why the hair on the left side of his face?

(d) What might be done to help him?

48 (a) What is the appearance of these hands caused by?

(b) What is the condition?

(c) Where does it proceed?

(d) What are the stages that occur?

(e) What treatment is available?

48

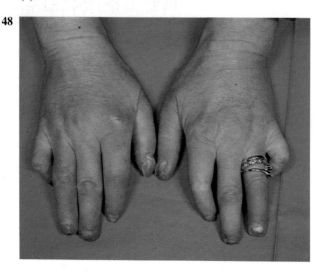

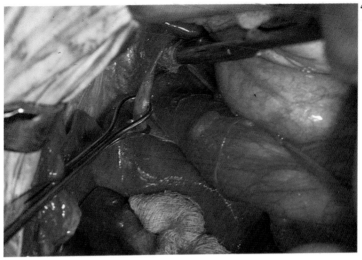

49 (a) What type of upper abdominal operation is shown?
(b) What are the clinical features?
(c) What other types of hernia occur?
(d) What operation is usually carried out?
(e) How successful is this?

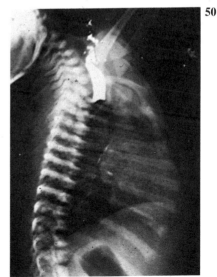

50 (a) A barium meal was done in this baby. What is shown?
(b) Prior to that, a catheter was passed down the oesophagus. Why?
(c) What are the various types of the condition?
(d) What are the clinical features?
(e) What surgery will be required?

51

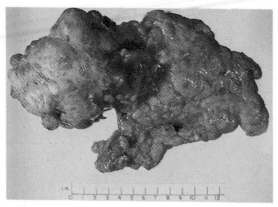

51 (a) What is this relatively rare tumour of the stomach?
(b) What areas of the stomach are usually involved?
(c) What characteristics may be found?
(d) What treatment is involved?

52 (a) What does this specimen show?
(b) What further investigations may be made?
(c) How common is this form of disease?
(d) What serious complication may arise?

52

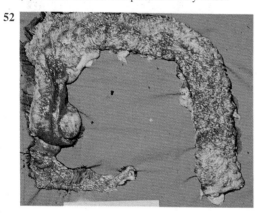

53 (a) What is the condition shown?
(b) What is the common symptom?
(c) How should this condition be investigated?
(d) What treatment is required?

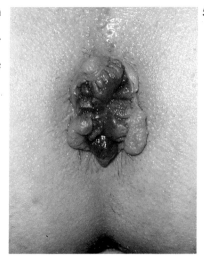

54 (a) What condition is shown here on arteriography?
(b) What is this caused by?
(c) What further problems may arise?
(d) How might these arise?
(e) What should be done?

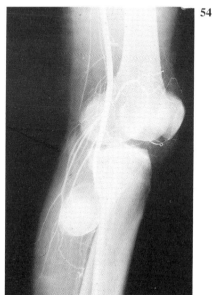

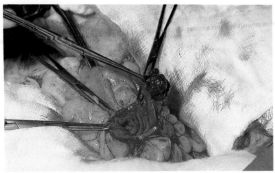

55 (a) What is visible here?
(b) Is it benign or malignant?
(c) What symptom would suggest the diagnosis?
(d) What two investigations are usually done?
(e) If in doubt, what other technique is used?

56 (a) Which two features does this specimen show?
(b) What would have been the reasons for the patient's operation?
(c) What is the follow-up?

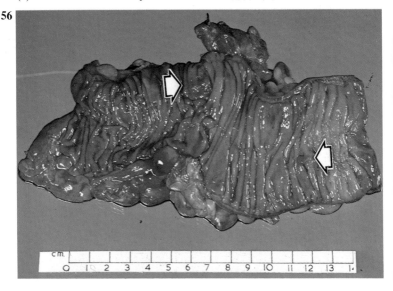

57 (a) What is shown?
(b) What is the main symptom?
(c) What other signs may occur?
(d) What investigations are done?
(e) What forms of treatment are available?

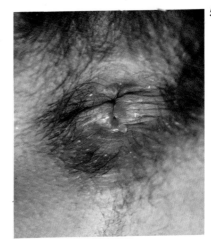

58 (a) What tumour involving the ileum is shown?
(b) How does it present in the patient?
(c) What treatment is required?
(d) Would you expect further trouble?

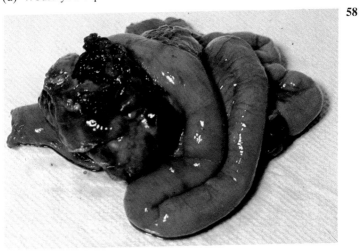

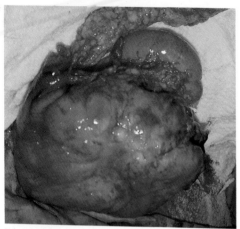

59 (a) This large mass was involving the gastric omentum. What might it be?
(b) What is its primary origin?
(c) What clinical features might be present?
(d) What treatment might be carried out?

60 (a) What is shown in this section of the liver?
(b) Which well known syndrome associated with the liver is this?
(c) What are the common sites of the primary lesion?
(d) What investigation should be carried out?
(e) What treatment is available?

61 (a) What is visible in the left thorax?
(b) How would this be manifested?
(c) How would you make the definitive diagnosis?
(d) Which types of the condition are these?
(e) How would this be dealt with?

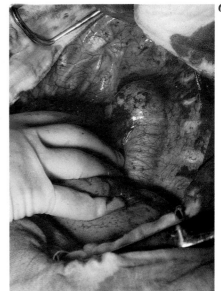

62 (a) What do these arteriograms show?
(b) What symptomatology was present prior to operation?
(c) What treatment was involved?
(d) What other treatment may be used?

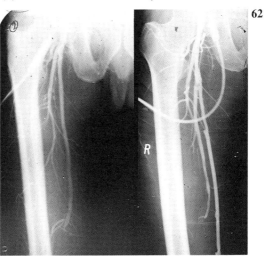

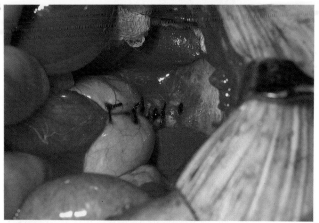

63 (a) What upper abdominal operation is shown? What is the procedure?
(b) What symptoms would have been present?
(c) What is the rationale of the operation?

64 (a) What is shown here?
(b) How does this happen?
(c) What symptoms may indicate the problem?
(d) What treatment is necessary?

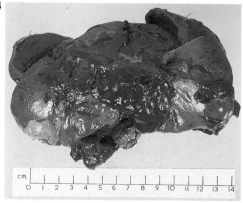

65 (a) What is obvious here?
(b) What treatment might have saved the organ and controlled the bleeding?
(c) Sutures may fail, what else might help?

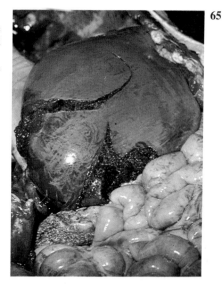

66 (a) What is shown here?
(b) What could produce this?
(c) What symptoms were present?
(d) What treatment is required?

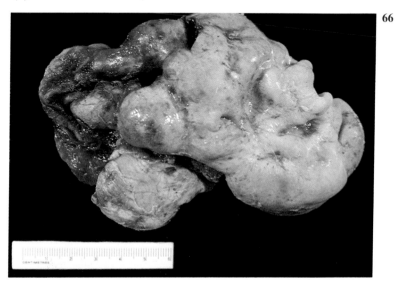

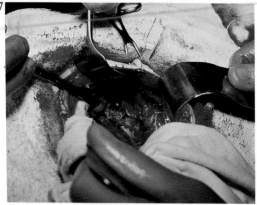

67 (a) A sudden severe injury of the lower abdomen. What is this?
(b) What conditions produce this?
(c) What are the clinical features?
(d) What treatment would be used?

68 (a) What is the problem here?
(b) How would this happen?
(c) What might a plain X-ray show?
(d) How would this condition be dealt with?

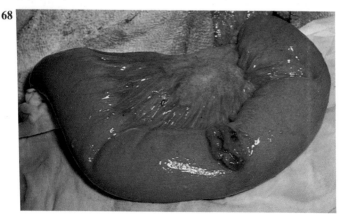

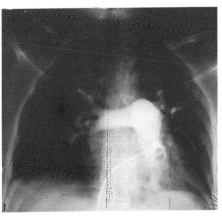

69 (a) What does this angiogram show?
(b) What condition is present?
(c) How has this occurred?
(d) What treatment is required?
(e) What was the result in this case?

70 (a) What is seen here?
(b) What causes this?
(c) How would you localise the area?
(d) What other discharges occur from the nipple?
(e) What do these discharges suggest?

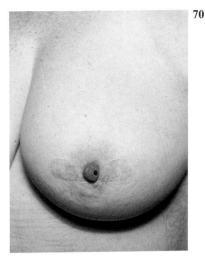

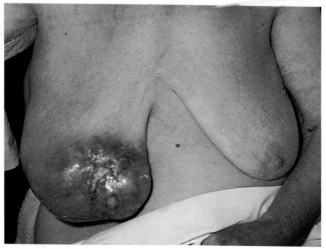

71 (a) What lesion is present in the right breast here?
(b) Is this condition malignant?
(c) What is the benign part?
(d) How would you deal with it?

72 (a) What is this lesion?
(b) What changes have taken place in the breast as a result of this?
(c) Is it purely an eczematous reaction?
(d) What lies behind the areola?

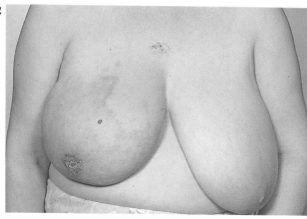

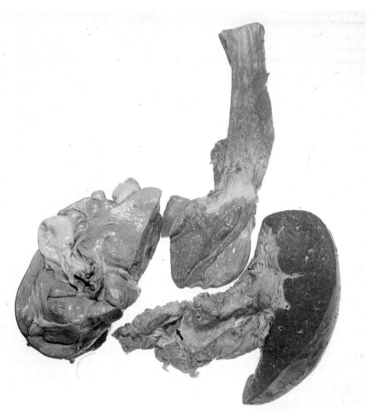

73 (a) What does this picture show?
(b) What is the primary cause?
(c) What is the problem with oesophageal varices and what help can be given?
(d) What results from this liver problem?
(e) What treatment is required for a reasonable outcome?

74

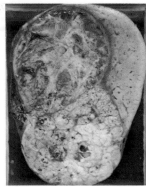

74 (a) A 22-month-old baby presented with a huge mass in the right hypochondrium. What is the diagnosis?
(b) What investigations could be done?
(c) What treatment was required?
(d) What future would the baby have?

75

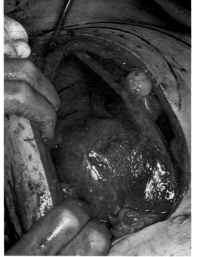

75 (a) What problem is present in this 5-year-old girl?
(b) What are the symptoms?
(c) What tests should be done?
(d) What operation should be done?

76 (a) What is the diagnosis of this lesion shown on barium?
(b) How common is this?
(c) What is the commonest tumour of this area?
(d) What other tumours may affect this area?
(e) What operation should be done?

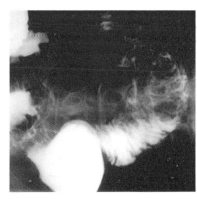

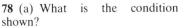

77 (a) What is the diagnosis of this lesion?
(b) How common is it?
(c) Is it seen in the circumcised?
(d) What is the type of tumour?
(e) What is the treatment?

78 (a) What is the condition shown?
(b) What was the preliminary condition?
(c) What organisms are involved?
(d) What treatment is required?

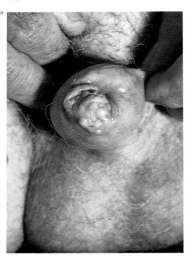

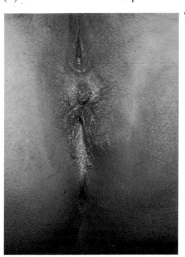

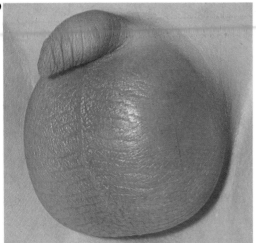

79 (a) A young boy had a sudden onset of lower abdominal pain and tenderness in the scrotum. What has happened?
(b) Is inflammation in the scrotum common in children?
(c) On examination the cord was thickened. What particular diagnosis does this support?
(d) What treatment should be instituted?
(e) What about the right testicle?

80 (a) At operation these objects were seen, what are they?
(b) What causes them?
(c) What are the definitive hosts?
(d) What change is there in the blood?
(e) Where are these objects found in the body?
(f) What tests establish diagnosis?

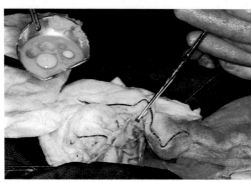

81 (a) What respiratory problem is present?
(b) What are the primary causes of this?
(c) What is its effect?
(d) What other effect is related?
(e) How can the chest be cleared?

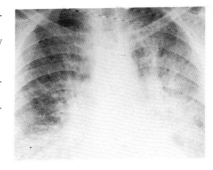

82 (a) What is shown in the left ureter and what is its composition?
(b) What symptoms may be present?
(c) What investigations will help?
(d) What forms of management are there?

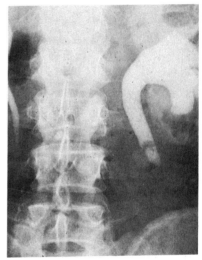

83 (a) What is probable diagnosis of this?
(b) What type of people are most susceptible to this?
(c) How should this be treated?
(d) What will happen in this patient?

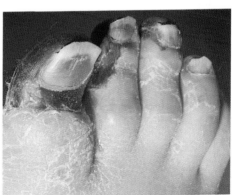

84

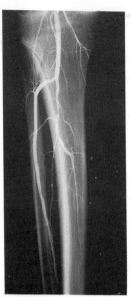

84 (a) What does this arteriogram show?
(b) What vessels are involved?
(c) What further disorder would be serious?
(d) How would this be diagnosed?

85

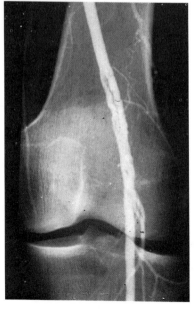

85 (a) What can be seen in this arteriogram?
(b) What might be the cause?
(c) What treatment can be done?
(d) What investigations should be carried out?

86 (a) What does this arteriogram show?
(b) What symptom could occur?
(c) Is any other vessel damaged?
(d) What operations could be done?

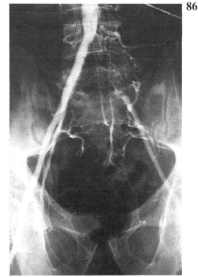

87 (a) This tumour was removed from the carotid artery region. What is it?
(b) What type of tumour is it?
(c) What investigation would be done?
(d) Where exactly is this tumour found?
(e) How is it dealt with?
(f) What dangers may arise at operation?

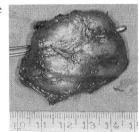

88 (a) What is shown on this picture?
(b) Why is it required?
(c) What are some of the causes of this condition?
(d) What can be done for emergency haematemesis?

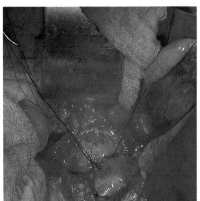

89

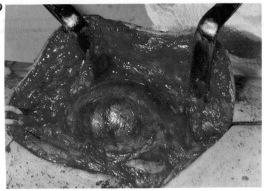

89 (a) What lesion is present in the wrist?
(b) How would it arise in this area?
(c) How should it be dealt with?

90 (a) What condition is being dealt with here?
(b) How does it present?
(c) What type of people get this problem?
(d) What operation is done?

90

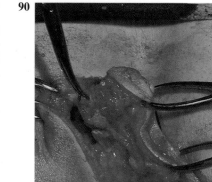

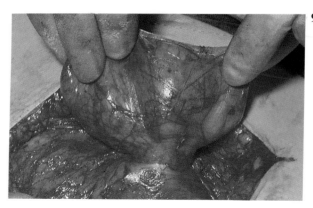

91 (a) The lesion is obvious but it has a special name, which is?
(b) What type of hernia is it?
(c) What is the main symptom?
(d) What sign may help in diagnosis?
(e) Is there any notable danger?

92 (a) What does this X-ray show?
(b) What term is often used for the condition?
(c) Which parts of the body may be involved?
(d) What type occupations cause most trouble with the condition?
(e) What are the clinical features?
(f) How can it be treated?

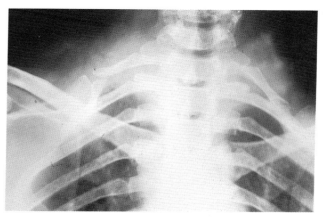

93

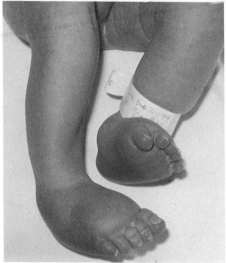

93 (a) What is wrong with this baby?
(b) The condition was present very early in life. What does this suggest?
(c) Which sex is usually involved?
(d) What complications may arise in the future?
(e) What treatment may be used?

94

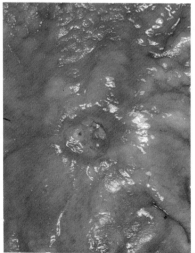

94 (a) What is evident here?
(b) Is there a significant area in the ulcer?
(c) What was done for this?
(d) What investigation of the ulcer should be done?

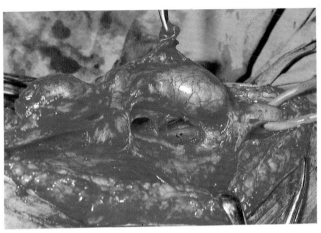

95 (a) What is the problem in this 24-year-old woman?
(b) There was no obvious disease process. What can be concluded?
(c) What further investigation should be done?
(d) What is the treatment?

96 (a) What is obvious in the abdomen of this man?
(b) What else is present?
(c) What are the causes of the above?
(d) What is probably the best type of suturing to prevent the condition?

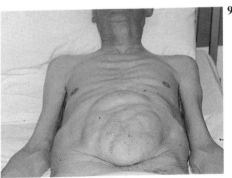

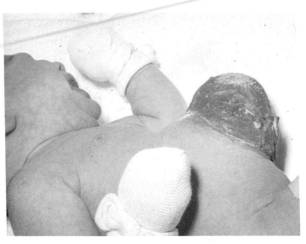

97 (a) What condition is present?
(b) What problems are there?
(c) What treatment may be carried out?
(d) In the case of a very large protrusion, what more may be done?

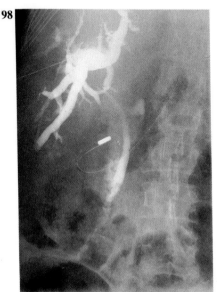

98 (a) What does this cholangiogram illustrate?
(b) What is the possible cause?
(c) What clinical features may be present?
(d) What investigations are helpful?
(e) What treatment may be helpful?
(f) What is the prognosis?

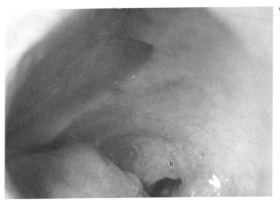

99 (a) What does the dusky pigmentation of the skin seen here suggest?
(b) Where else might this pigmentation be noticed?
(c) What treatment should be given?
(d) What tests would confirm the diagnosis?

100 (a) What condition does this autopsy display?
(b) How does it present?
(c) What are the clinical features?
(d) What treatment should be given?
(e) What problem is difficult to overcome?
(f) What has caused this problem?

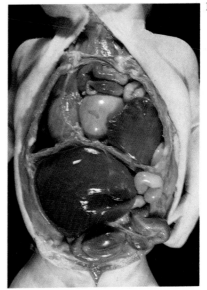

101

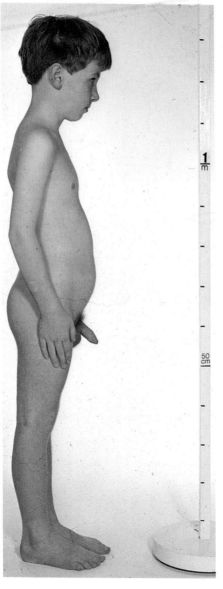

101 (a) What condition does this 7-year-old boy show? What does it denote?
(b) What causes this and usually from which condition?
(c) What other conditions produce this problem?
(d) How is diagnosis finally decided?
(e) What does the dexamethasone suppression test do?

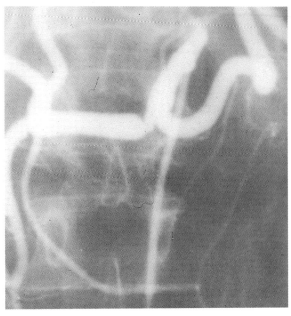

102 (a) What does this arteriogram show?
(b) What may be the cause?
(c) What are the clinical features?
(d) What treatment is effective?

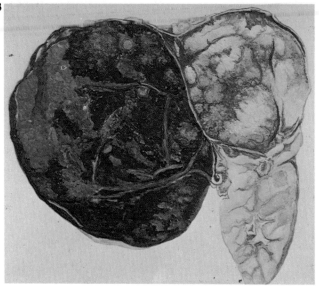

103 (a) What is this tumour of the neural crest and what is the origin?
(b) In which decade of life is the tumour often found?
(c) Does it metastasise?
(d) What are the clinical features?
(e) What treatment is required?

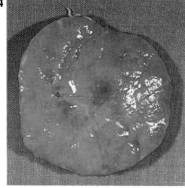

104 (a) What is this tumour which was removed from above the kidney?
(b) What clinical features may be present?
(c) How would you diagnose this condition?
(d) How may the tumour be observed?

105 (a) This patient has typical features of what condition?
(b) What are these features?
(c) What produces these features?
(d) What other changes may be present?

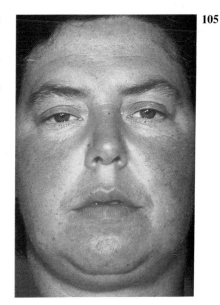

106 (a) What is this endocrine tumour?
(b) What clinical features may be present?
(c) What is causing the problems?
(d) Would radiology be of help in the diagnosis?
(e) What is the main treatment?

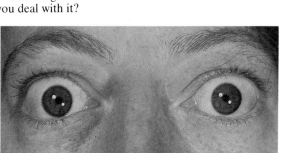

107 (a) What is evident in this patient?
(b) What are the clinical signs?
(c) How would you deal with it?

108

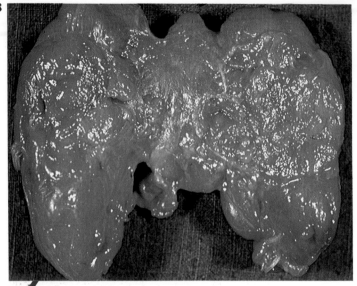

108 (a) This is a section of which gland?
(b) What was the operation done for?
(c) What preparations were made for surgery?
(d) What surgery was done?

109

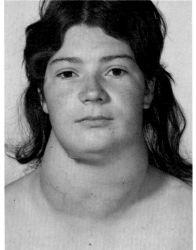

109 (a) What is this condition?
(b) What are causes of this?
(c) What problems may arise from the swelling?
(d) What types of gland changes are there?
(e) Should surgery be done?

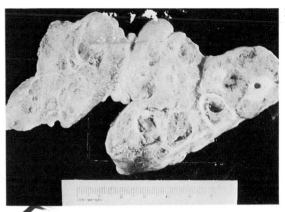

110

110 (a) What is evident in this cross-section of a thyroid?
(b) What is the cause of colloid goitre?
(c) What would make you become suspicious of cancer?
(d) What sex is more likely to develop cancer of the thyroid?

111 (a) What is the obvious swelling in this elderly woman?
(b) What is the cause?
(c) How would you rule out cancer in the elderly?
(d) What is often visible in a large goitre?
(e) Why is surgery performed?

111

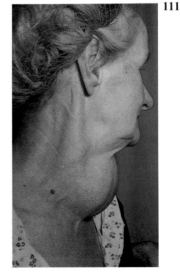

57

112

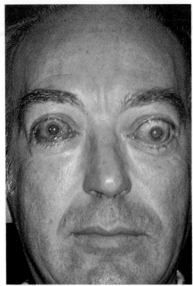

112 (a) What is this distressing but fortunately rare condition?
(b) What medical treatment may help for a time?
(c) What clinical features may be present?
(d) What surgery can help?

1

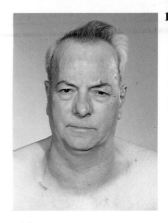

113 (a) What may this lesion be?
(b) In which sex is it more common?
(c) Is it a slowly growing lesion?
(d) Where are the sites of metastasis?
(e) What is the obvious treatment?
(f) Would radioiodine help?

114

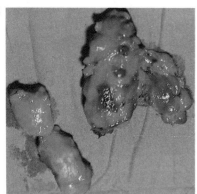

114 (a) These glands were excised from the neck of a young man. What is the condition?
(b) What operation has been performed?
(c) How common is this tumour?
(d) How may it be spotted?
(e) What is its rate of progress?

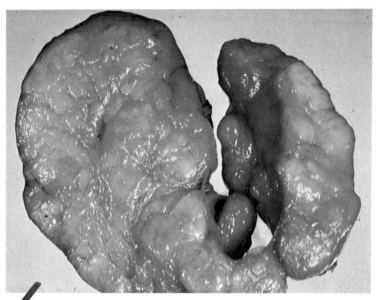

115 (a) What is the diagnosis of this gland?
(b) What type of condition is this?
(c) What treatment is used?
(d) How is the diagnosis confirmed?

116 (a) This patient has a rare condition in which the thyroid feels like hard wood. What might it be?
(b) What other diagnosis would you expect?
(c) How would the diagnosis be confirmed?
(d) What danger may the condition present?
(e) What treatment may help?

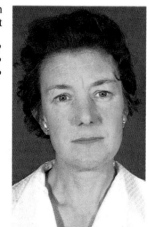

117

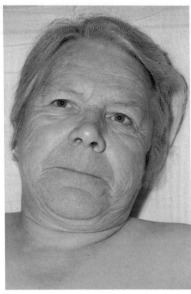

117 (a) What signs does this woman have?
(b) What might be the diagnosis?
(c) How would you confirm this?
(d) What are the dangers of this condition?
(e) What should be done to help?

118

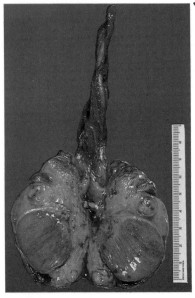

118 (a) What do you see in this specimen?
(b) What is the likely diagnosis?
(c) What should be remembered regarding swellings in this area?
(d) What investigations would be done?
(e) How would this problem be treated?

119 (a) What type of testicular tumour is shown?
(b) How is it classified?
(c) What is the most dangerous type?
(d) What chemotherapy may be used?

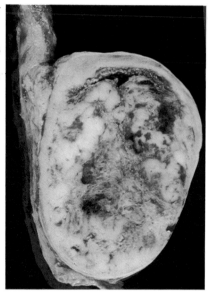

119

120 (a) A 36-year-old man noted a swelling in the left side of his scrotum. What is the diagnosis?
(b) What would confirm the diagnosis?
(c) What would indicate a serious problem?
(d) What other indices may be of value?
(e) What treatment may be given?

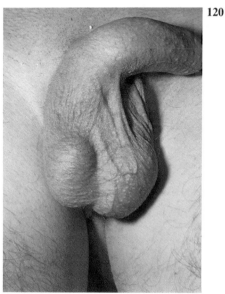

120

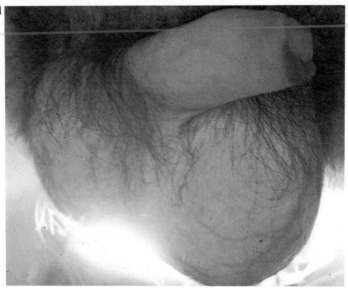

121 (a) What is present in this scrotum?
(b) How often does the processus vaginalis stay open?
(c) In children, how often is the bowel down in the scrotum?
(d) What distinguishes communicating hydroceles?

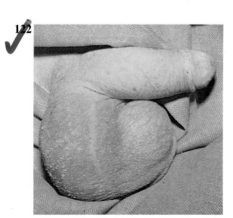

122 (a) What is this condition likely to be?
(b) Where does the infection come from?
(c) What are the early features?
(d) What is Prehn's sign?
(e) How can you differentiate this condition from torsion of the testis?

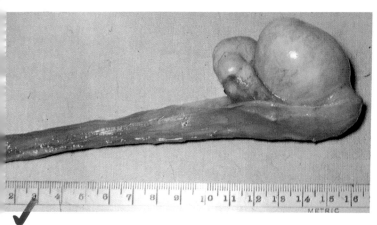

123 (a) What is shown here?
(b) What is the diagnosis?
(c) What would make its presence be suspected?
(d) What investigation is especially helpful in diagnosis?

124 (a) What does this pathological specimen show?
(b) What is the likely cause?
(c) When was the diagnosis made in this case?
(d) What investigations would have helped to make the diagnosis previously?

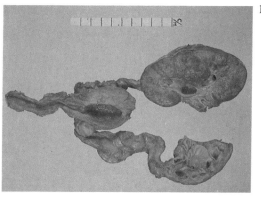

125

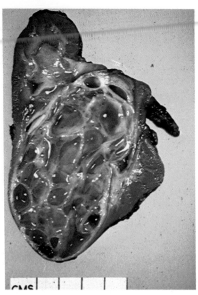

125 (a) What condition is present?
(b) At what age and how does it present?
(c) What sign helps in the diagnosis?
(d) How is the diagnosis confirmed?
(e) What symptoms indicate the problem?
(f) If it is bilateral, what might be done?

126 (a) This patient developed a large mobile mass in the left side of her abdomen. What is the probable diagnosis?
(b) What investigations would be preferred?
(c) What would these show?
(d) What would the diagnosis and treatment be?

126

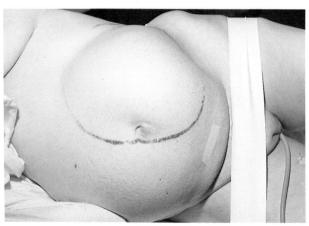

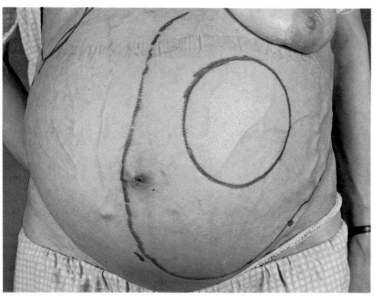

127 (a) What is the most likely cause of this mass?
(b) What do the blue lines indicate?
(c) What are the main causes of this condition?
(d) How could diagnosis be made?

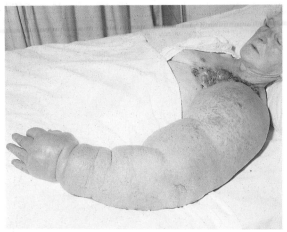

128 (a) This picture shows a rather florid condition. What is it?
(b) What is said to be the cause?
(c) What else do you observe?
(d) Would radiotherapy help?

129 (a) What is shown?
(b) What pathology is present?
(c) What type of tumour may be present?
(d) What was the previous primary tumour?

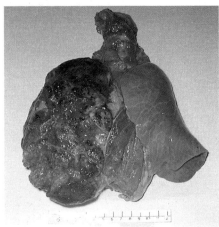

130 (a) What is shown here?
(b) What pathology is present?
(c) Where does the metastasis occur?
(d) What treatment may be given?

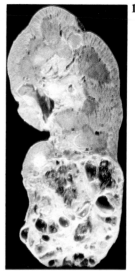

131 (a) This 8-year-old boy is pale and listless and has a mass in the left loin. What is the diagnosis?
(b) What are the clinical findings?
(c) How would the final diagnosis be made?
(d) What is the appearance of the lesion?

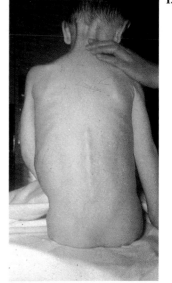

132

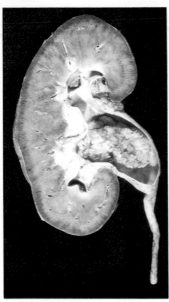

132 (a) A kidney specimen has been opened. What is shown?
(b) What would have alerted the clinician to the problem?
(c) What would the IVP have shown?
(d) What operation should be done?

133

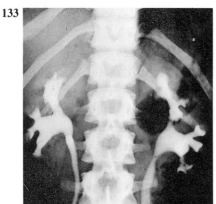

133 (a) What does this IVP show?
(b) What is the likely diagnosis?
(c) What test may support this?
(d) What symptoms may be present?
(e) What more specific investigation should be done?
(f) If the upper calyx only is involved and there are no signs elsewhere, what can be done?

134 (a) What is the diagnosis of this specimen?
(b) What are the features?
(c) What is present in the lower pole of the kidney?
(d) Why was nephrectomy done?

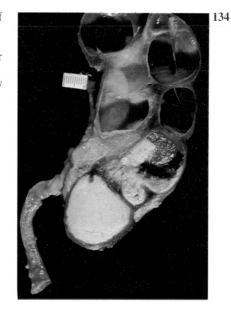

134

135 (a) What symptoms cause this kidney to be removed?
(b) What was the most likely cause?
(c) What tests would confirm this?
(d) What other investigations could be done?

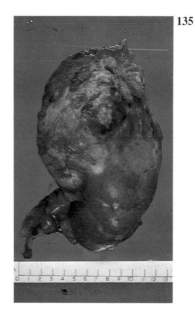

135

136

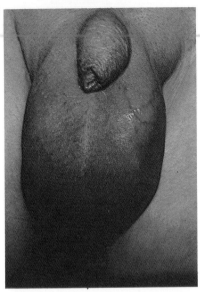

136 (a) What do you think has happened here?
(b) What does the redness above the scrotum suggest?
(c) What are the causes of urethral injuries?
(d) What investigation may be done?
(e) What treatment may be necessary?

137

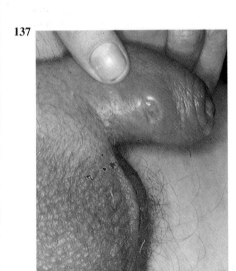

137 (a) The patient had a *stricture of the urethra* with retention of urine. What could be done to relieve him?
(b) What further should be done?
(c) After 2 weeks an abscess developed, leaving a shallow ulcer. What tests are required?
(d) What might underlie the cause of the problem?
(e) What are other causes of stricture of the urethra?
(f) What further investigations may be done?

138 (a) What is this lesion in the chest?
(b) What is the cause of this?
(c) Where does this happen?
(d) What is the main cause?
(e) What investigations are carried out?
(f) What does Type A and B reflect in terms of surgery?

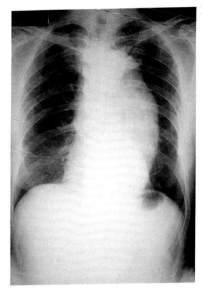

139 (a) What is wrong here?
(b) What investigation should be done?
(c) Should hormones be used?
(d) If they do not come down, what is done?
(e) Would you expect full potency?

140 (a) What is the difference between the two parts of the scrotum shown?
(b) What is the diagnosis?
(c) How does this condition develop?
(d) On which side is it more common, and why?
(e) What treatment should be done?

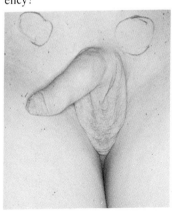

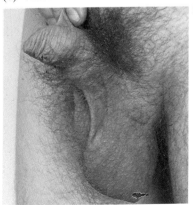

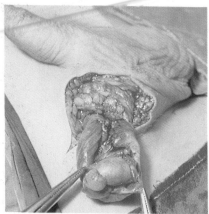

141 (a) An operation has been started. What is being done?
(b) What can be observed?
(c) When do the testicles normally descend into the scrotum?
(d) Why not leave the testicle in the inguinal canal?
(e) If there are bilateral undescended testes, when should the testes be fixed in the scrotum?

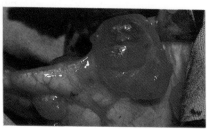

142 (a) What operation is this and what can be seen?
(b) What is the cause of these?
(c) What is the danger in these cases?
(d) How should this be treated?

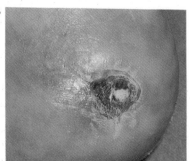

143 (a) What is visible here?
(b) What causes this?
(c) What clinical investigations may be done?
(d) What is the main investigation?
(e) How can blood flow be improved?

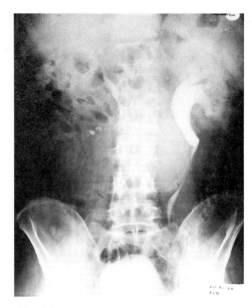

144 (a) What is shown in this IVP?
(b) What has caused this?
(c) What is the mass present?
(d) Why was an IVP done?
(e) What is the danger of IVP?

145 (a) What is seen in this X-ray?
(b) What conditions might result?
(c) What investigations may be done?
(d) In a general surgical unit, what is the most likely diagnosis?

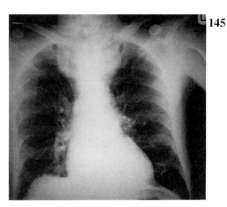

146

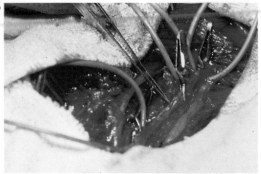

146 (a) An emergency operation. What might be the cause and what vessel was involved?
(b) How was it treated?
(c) What structures might be damaged in the area?
(d) What problems may arise in the post-operative period?

147

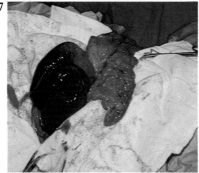

147 (a) What is the obvious problem in this abdomen?
(b) What clinical features would be present?
(c) What would you expect to find at operation?
(d) How would this be managed?
(e) How would you prevent a reoccurrence?

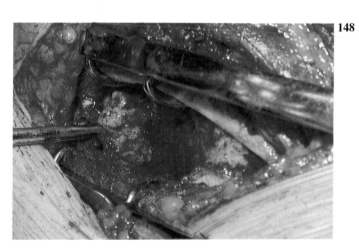

148 (a) What lesion is seen here in the chest?
(b) What other tumours may be present in the lung?
(c) What types of sarcoma are there in the pleural cavity?
(d) What treatment may be undertaken?

149 (a) What operation was done and what were the results?
(b) Why did this occur?
(c) How can this be prevented?
(d) What investigations might be made?
(e) In the past, what was done?

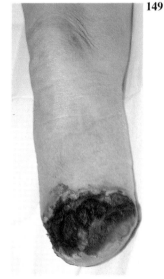

150 (a) What is the technique being used?
(b) What do the colours represent?
(c) What are the representative blood flows in this case?
(d) What does the lower figure indicate?

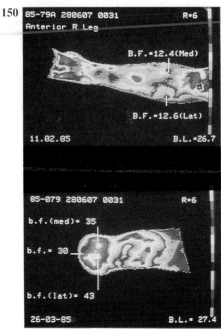

151 (a) What is shown here?
(b) How is this foot assessed?
(c) What can be done?
(d) How would treatment be chosen?

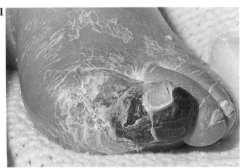

152 (a) What is shown in this operation in the neck?
(b) In which age group do these usually occur?
(c) What are the clinical features?
(d) What examination is carried out before operation?
(e) Where does this originate?

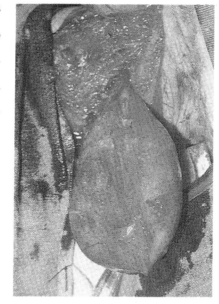

153 (a) What is shown here?
(b) What then is the diagnosis?
(c) What clinical features could be present?
(d) What treatment would be carried out?

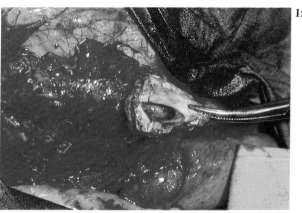

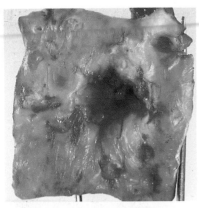

154 (a) What can be seen in this portion of the aorta?
(b) What clinical symptoms might be present?
(c) What is characteristic of this?
(d) How would the clinical diagnosis be established?
(e) What operative procedures would be helpful?

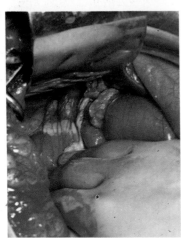

155 (a) What do the white areas here suggest in the upper abdomen?
(b) What is the symptomatology of this lesion?
(c) What are the causes of the disease?
(d) What investigations are carried out to establish the diagnosis?

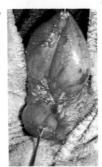

156 (a) What is this rare lesion present in the upper abdomen?
(b) How may it be demonstrated?
(c) How should it be treated?
(d) Why not divide the pancreas and release the obstruction?

157 (a) What is shown?
(b) What else is present?
(c) How can these be dealt with? What is the preferable method?

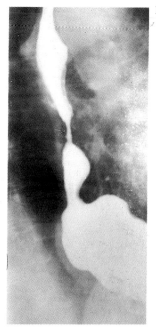

157

158 (a) What operation has been done?
(b) How would this condition present?
(c) What is the sex relationship of this condition?
(d) What is the problem in diagnosis?

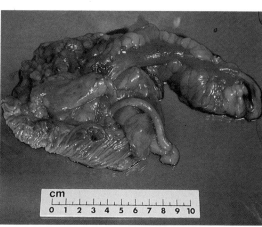

158

159

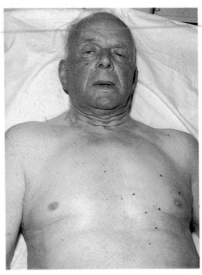

159 (a) What would be your first diagnosis in an elderly man with progressive jaundice?
(b) What are the characteristic features?
(c) What investigations would you carry out?
(d) How should it be treated?
(e) What is the prognosis?

160 (a) What is this discoloration of the abdomen called?
(b) What is the cause of it?
(c) What produces the greenish colour?
(d) What other sign is present on the abdominal skin?

160

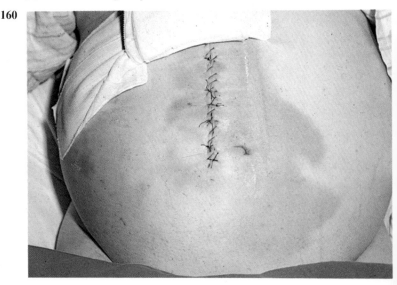

161 (a) What is seen here?
(b) What problems can arise?
(c) What is the main cause?
(d) How can this be dealt with urgently?
(e) What later treatment is helpful?

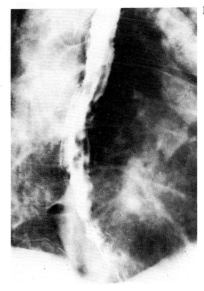

161

162 (a) What is seen in this film?
(b) Why is the mass so dark?
(c) What then is the diagnosis?
(d) What should be done?
(e) What might happen if it is left alone?

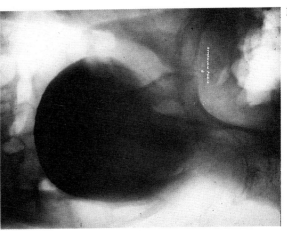

162

163

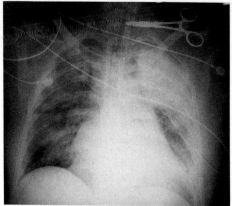

163 (a) What is seen in this X-ray from a patient in a critical care unit?
(b) What is the diagnosis?
(c) What is this condition?
(d) What is normally seen on X-ray?

164 (a) What is the injury sustained?
(b) What can be done?
(c) What are the problems that cause trouble?
(d) What can be done with the aortic lesion?

164

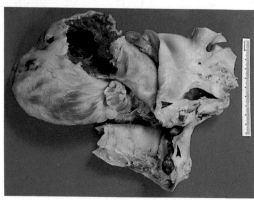

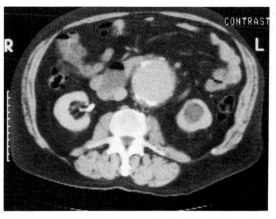

165 (a) A 75-year-old man had abdominal pain. What does the CT scan show?
(b) What further investigation may be done?
(c) What are the complications of this type of condition?
(d) What operations should be done?

166 (a) What is present on the right side of the picture?
(b) How may this develop?
(c) What type of trauma would produce this?
(d) How can you indicate the type of bowel present?

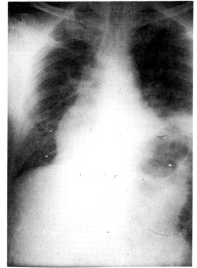

167

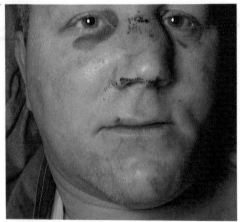

167 (a) What has happened to this man?
(b) What are the main features?
(c) How would this problem be treated?
(d) What about the deviated septum?
(e) What other problem could occur?

168 (a) What injury has this patient sustained?
(b) Is it easy to diagnose this clinically?
(c) What treatment is necessary?
(d) Are there any further problems?

168

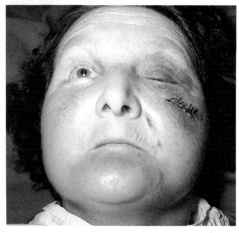

169 (a) This is a very severe facial injury. What has happened?
(b) What would cause this?
(c) What name is given to this group of injuries?
(d) What treatment may be required?

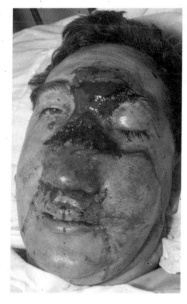

170 (a) What is the swelling in the chest due to?
(b) What type of the condition is this likely to be?
(c) How is this diagnosed?
(d) How would you assess the problem?
(e) If the patient is suitable and the problem is critical, what should be done?

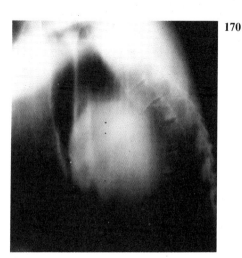

171

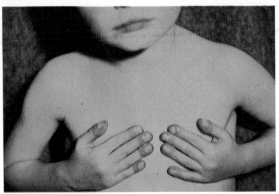

171 (a) What diagnosis would seem to fit this young boy?
(b) What are the four problem areas?
(c) Is it possible to save the child and if so, how?
(d) What are the clinical features?
(e) What are the results of surgery?

172 (a) Barium has been swallowed. What does it show?
(b) What is the probable cause?
(c) What name is given to this?
(d) What are the clinical features?
(e) What treatment is required?

172

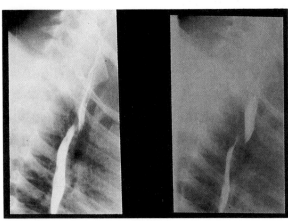

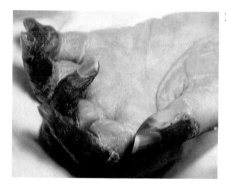

173 (a) What is present?
(b) How did this develop?
(c) What else would give such a serious problem?
(d) What should have been done?
(e) What would follow after that?

174 (a) A previous vascular operation has been done, now there is a pulsatile swelling. What may have occurred?
(b) Why should this occur?
(c) What is there a risk of?
(d) How may the condition be dealt with?
(e) What else might be done?

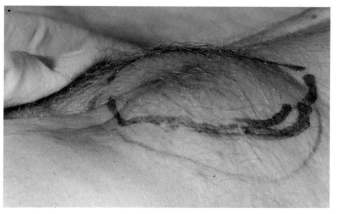

175

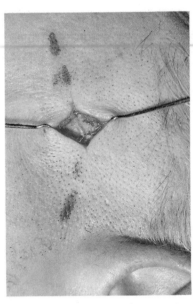

175 (a) What operation is being carried out?
(b) Why is it being done?
(c) What are the symptoms?
(d) Is it purely localised to the area?
(e) What is another name for the condition and what age group does it affect?
(f) What therapy may help?

176

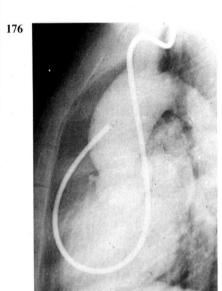

176 (a) What lesion is shown here by angiocardiography?
(b) What are the symptoms?
(c) What other clinical features may be present?
(d) What types of the condition are possible?

177 (a) What lesion is under repair?
(b) What types of these are possible?
(c) What signs suggest a secundum defect?
(d) What is the problem with the atrio-ventricular canal defect?

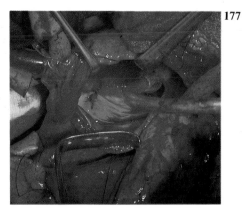

177

178 (a) What condition does this show?
(b) What are the symptoms?
(c) What is seen in cardio-angiography?
(d) What signs may aid in diagnosis?

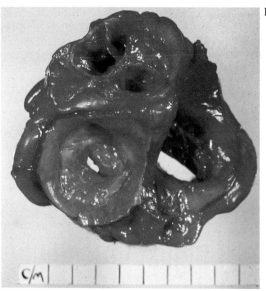

178

179

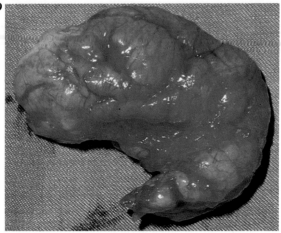

179 (a) What is this swelling which was removed from the oesophagus?
(b) How may it present?
(c) How common is it?
(d) How are these detected?
(e) What operation would be done for treatment?

180 (a) What is this lesion in the popliteal artery?
(b) What symptoms would make the patient aware of this?
(c) What investigation should be carried out?
(d) What treatment is required?

180

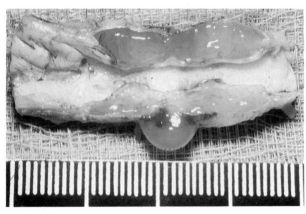

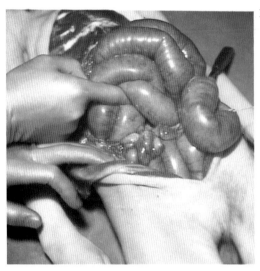

181 (a) What problem is shown by this post-mortem examination?

(b) What clinical features should have alerted a doctor?

(c) What would have saved this life?

(d) What incident might have been the cause of death?

182 (a) What operation has been done?

(b) Is this a common way of doing the operation?

(c) What is done usually?

(d) Why the difference?

(e) What is done if the iliac area is thrombosed or severely blocked with atheroma?

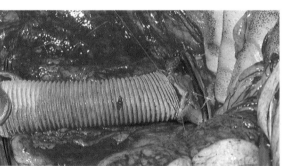

183

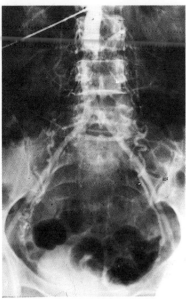

183 (a) What is shown on this X-ray?
(b) What may be the cause of this?
(c) What treatment would be done if this were thrombosis only?
(d) What stops this treatment and necessitates an operation?
(e) What clinical sign would have alerted the doctor that such a block was present?

184 (a) What condition is present in the small bowel here?
(b) What then might be the diagnosis, and why?
(c) What might the primary site be and what other condition might be thought of?
(d) How common is the disease shown and what symptoms may be present?

184

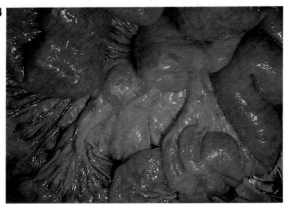

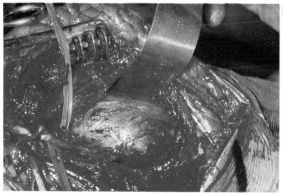

185 (a) What is this lesion?
(b) What is its type?
(c) What are its causes?
(d) What is the most likely complication?
(e) How would this case be dealt with?

186 (a) What is shown here?
(b) What is this done for?
(c) What vessels are affected?
(d) Is the operation absolutely necessary?
(e) What procedure is done?

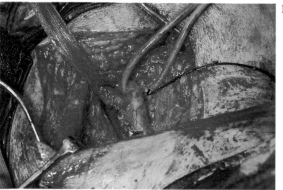

187

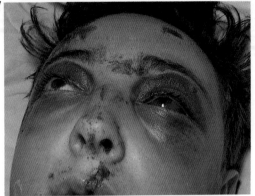

187 (a) What injury is shown?
(b) What may result from this?
(c) What investigations may help?
(d) What index is used to indicate the patient's status?
(e) What are the parts of this index?

188 (a) What does this appear to be?
(b) What cysts occur in this area?
(c) How may types of cysts be differentiated?
(d) What complication may arise?
(e) What may happen in babies with the condition shown?

188

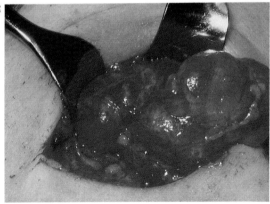

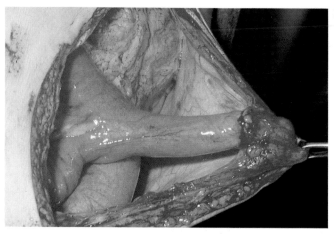

189 (a) What is illustrated at this operation?
(b) If the attachment went so far as to discharge material, what would it be called?
(c) What major problem may occur?
(d) What other problems may arise?

190 (a) What is the name given to this condition?
(b) What is the description?
(c) What is difference between this and an atheroma?
(d) What type of people get this problem?
(e) What investigation shows up the problem?
(f) What treatment is advised?

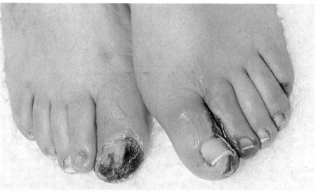

190

191 (a) What problem is present here?
(b) How has this taken place?
(c) What is another cause of this?
(d) What problems may arise in the patient?

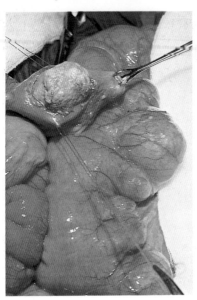

192 (a) What is the problem in this tongue?
(b) Is this serious?
(c) What treatment should be given?
(d) What is the risk of involvement of the lymph nodes?

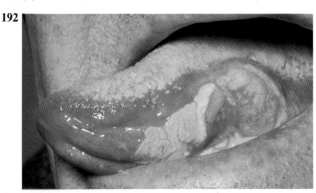

193 (a) What is shown here on barium meal?
(b) What symptom suggests this?
(c) How can you be sure it is not just a previous ulcer?
(d) What other investigations should be done?
(e) Why should these be done?

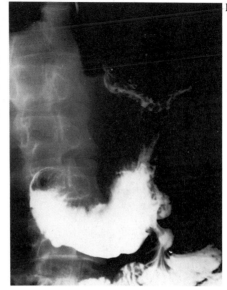

193

194 (a) What is this lesion in the umbilicus?
(b) What specific name is given to it?
(c) Why was it thus named?
(d) What treatment is given?

194

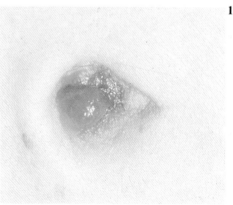

195

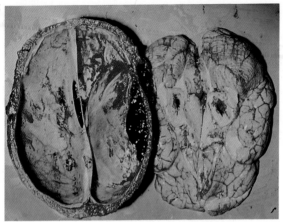

195 (a) How would you define this lesion?
(b) What damage had been sustained?
(c) Which vessel is most likely to be damaged?
(d) What follows after the bleeding?
(e) What is the mortality rate? Why?

196 (a) This woman had an abdominal operation. What is present in the leg and what may have preceded it?
(b) What are the common ovarian malignant tumours?
(c) What other types of malignant disease may affect the ovary?
(d) Are these tumours easily noticed?
(e) How are the tumours recognised?

196

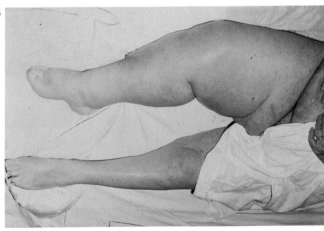

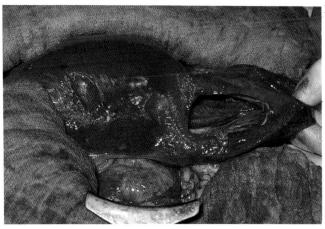

197 (a) What is seen in this upper abdominal operation?
(b) How can this condition present in the liver?
(c) In the multiple case, what else may be present?
(d) How should the condition be dealt with?
(e) What should be looked out for?

198 (a) This patient was assaulted. What injuries are present?
(b) How are these injuries confirmed?
(c) What clinical features are present to increase the problems?
(d) What other problems may arise?
(e) How are the injuries stabilised?

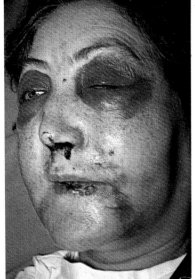

199

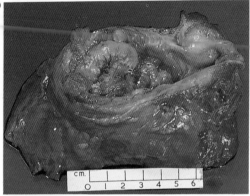

199 (a) What organ is shown and what is wrong with it?
(b) What is the sex ratio of this condition?
(c) What type of lesion is present?
(d) What are the clinical features?
(e) How is the lesion diagnosed?
(f) What is the treatment?

200

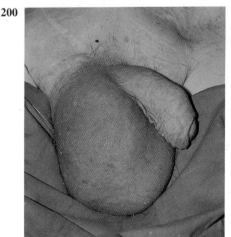

200 (a) What does this swelling suggest?
(b) On examination, the testis lay in front and was normal, but the epididymis was hard. What does this suggest?
(c) What would section of the scrotal contents show?
(d) What is this rare pathology?

ANSWERS

1 (a) *Peau d'orange* is evidence of *cancer of the breast*.
  b) The pits are the openings of the fixed sweat ducts that cannot expand with the oedema.
  c) Chest X-ray, needle biopsy, and axillary node biopsy.
  d) (i) Excision of the tumour plus irradiation of the whole breast, with extra radiation of the tumour site.
  (ii) Lumpectomy and axillary clearance of the nodes and radiotherapy to the axilla.
  (iii) Simple mastectomy, ± deep X-ray therapy (DXT) or tamoxifen if a hormone-responsive tumour.
  e) Tamoxifen with mastectomy if the tumour increases.
  f) Do the mastectomy at the second, i.e. progesterone, stage of hormones.

2 (a) *Skin necrosis following carbuncle.*
  b) Debridement of slough is required. Antibiotics are usually used for staphylococcus, but a swab for bacteriology is needed.
  c) Poorly controlled diabetes.
  d) Skin grafting.

3 (a) Swelling at the tip with dark black areas and bleeding.
  b) Trauma to the lesion, which may have begun as a seborrhoeic wart.
  c) Biopsy. This was found to be a *malignant melanoma*.
  d) Excision of big toe. No glands were noted in groin region.
  e) Melanoma is commonest on the trunk and the leg.
  f) Thickness of the primary tumour (Breslow).
  g) Dacarbazine, vincristine.

4 (a) Gas in tissues of the upper thigh.
  b) Gas gangrene is caused by war injuries; civilian trauma, as in this case of a gunshot wound; and surgery, especially in relation to the colon and biliary tract.
  c) *Clostridium welchii* (the commonest), *C. oedematiens* or *C. septicum.*
  d) First surgery to open the areas and excise the damaged tissues, then hyperbaric oxygen and penicillin or metronidazole.

5 (a) A cellulitis of the lower eyelid, with pus evident.
  b) By spreading from the maxilla; the cause may be related to the mother.
  c) X-ray of the maxilla and culture of the pus.
  d) The spread of the infection to the eye, meninges or cavernous sinus.
  e) Antibiotics.

6 (a) Bloody diarrhoea involving the rectum and colon.
  b) Ischaemic colitis, infective colitis or Crohn's disease.
  c) By endoscopy, biopsy or barium enema.
  d) Drug therapy with salicylates, mesalazine, or osalozine. Corticosteroid foams where the disease is local and corticosteroid enemas for extensive areas. Cyclosporins may be tried.
  e) Ileostomy and mucous fistula in the distal colon; or subtotal or total colectomy.

7 (a) *Ludwig's angina.*
(b) Under the deep cervical fascia.
(c) Gross swelling may give rise to elevation of the tongue, producing oral obstruction.
(d) Usually staphylococcus, but may be streptococcus.
(e) If anaesthetic is used, it must be well controlled as the trachea may be obstructed.

8 (a) Either dried blood or a dangerous process is present.
(b) Yes. This ulcer may be a lesion of *anthrax.*
(c) From carrying sacks of bone meal on the shoulder if there is irritation of the skin when anthrax is present in the bone meal.
(d) Small vesicles round the ulcer, and enlarged lymph nodes.
(e) By investigating a smear of the fluid from a vesicle.

9 (a) Swelling of the right thumb, redness and the presence of lymphangitis.
(b) Usually from a prick or other damage to the thumb enabling penetration by organisms.
(c) *Tendon sheath infection,* which may be serious.
(d) Antibiotics. Note the presence of early necrosis of the skin. An incision may be needed to let out the pus.
(e) Stiffness of the thumb, affecting its mobility.

10 (a) One might suspect a neoplastic lesion but the rapidity of growth and ulceration suggests a *keratoacanthoma* (molluscum sebaceum).
(b) Cancer, but the process there was too rapid.
(c) A rapidly growing swelling of symmetrical shape with a keratin plug.
(d) The keratin is removed with a Volkmann's spoon and the clear area left behind gradually heals.

11 (a) The patient had toxaemia, with a rise in his temperature and pulse rate.
(b) Yes: he was a farmer.
(c) From contact with bone meal.
(d) *Anthrax adentis.*
(e) Other types of anthrax are the pulmonary form (wool sorter's disease) and the much less common alimentary form which resembles cholera.

12 (a) Fistula from the small bowel.
(b) A portion of ileum has been trapped in a hernia.
(c) *Richter's hernia.*
(d) The opening of the fistula is cleansed, a lower abdominal incision with resection of the fistula and anastomosis of the bowel is performed. Antibiotic cover is used.

13 (a) Possible leakage of blood indicating *rupture of a popliteal aneurysm.*
(b) A mass which may or may not pulsate.
(c) Arteriography showed a large mass behind the femur, indicating the popliteal aneurysm.
(d) Resection of the aneurysm, and a graft procedure related to the size of vessels.

14 (a) Haemorrhoidectomy.
(b) Bleeding, protrusion, mucus, general discomfort.
(c) Cancer of the rectum or colon, polyps, diverticular disease.
(d) Proctoscopy, sigmoidoscopy, and colonoscopy.
(e) The presence of third and fourth degree haemorrhoids.

15 (a) *An arteriovenous fistula.*
(b) The presence of a thrill over the swelling, distended veins, and a murmur.
(c) Angiography.

(d) Depending on the number of A–V connections, the veins could be tied off and the connections blocked by plugging, or the main artery could be removed and an alternative other artery or graft inserted.
(e) If the fistula is occluded on compression then the pulse rate will slow.

16 (a) Blockage of an artery by thrombosis or embolism.
(b) Arteriography, culture of the foot, and a test for diabetes.
(c) The fourth toe was excised but the trauma made matters worse.
(d) Thermography or isotope injections to determine the blood flow.
(e) It really depends on the arterial problem. If a long graft to the lower tibial vessels could be done, there is a chance of avoiding amputation.

17 (a) A typical *varicose ulcer,* related to the presence of incompetent large veins.
(b) The venous ulcer is typically oval and is present either on the malleolus or posterior to it.
(c) The venous pressure may be 40 mmHg or even greater.
(d) Deep vein thrombosis is probably the most important.

18 (a) A *gravitational ulcer* resulting from deep vein thrombosis.
(b) These ulcers have no definite shape, with one ulcerated area graduating into another.
(c) Oedema, which need not be of great extent, but the ulcer may be large and serpiginous.
(d) No. Varicose veins are absent unless already present prior to venous thrombosis.

19 (a) Risus sardonicus.
(b) Tetanus.
(c) General malaise, pyrexia, a rapid pulse rate. The following day, muscular spasms occurred, often in the facial muscles.
(d) In this case by a puncture in the side of the foot when playing barefoot.
(e) If immunised it should not occur. The treatment is not easy. Immune globulins are given to control spasms; anaesthesia or a drug such as Valium may be needed; curare may help the spasms; and penicillin is used to kill the organisms.

20 (a) A *typical squamous carcinoma*, no glands in the neck are involved.
(b) Under local anaesthesia, a W shape of wedge limits the extent of the lesion. The orbicularis muscle is excised with the cancer. The muscle is repaired and the mucosa and skin are repaired, making the W become a Y shape.
(c) Only if secondary recurrence.
(d) Very successful if no glandular involvement.

21 (a) An ulcer.
(b) Trauma, tubercle or tumour.
(c) Culture of the ulcer, a biopsy, and a chest radiograph.
(d) On the posterior third of the tongue.

22 (a) A cyst, an angioma, a tumour.
(b) By feel and by needle biopsy. The histology showed a *venous angioma*.
(c) Squamous cell cancer (95% of such tumours); lymphangioma; rhabdomyoma.
(d) Papilloma.
(e) By TNM (tumour, nodes and metastases) classification.

23 (a) *Basal cell carcinoma, i.e. a rodent ulcer.*
(b) A nodular lesion with the typical 'pearly' nodules.
(c) Not usually.
(d) Radiotherapy or excision.

24 (a) Because the swelling in the left side of the face is more evident.

(b) Pain in the left side of the face, especially in the upper tooth.

(c) Epistaxis from the left side of the nose.

(d) X-ray of the face showed an opaque view of the antrum and a biopsy confirmed a *squamous cancer of the left maxillary antrum.*

(e) By radiotherapy and partial or total maxillectomy.

25 (a) *Parotitis* with a possible abscess.

(b) Inspection of the opening of the parotid duct confirmed the presence of pus.

(c) Because a tight fascia is present over the gland.

(d) Much less now since dental hygiene has improved.

(e) Usually the elderly, dehydrated or debilitated.

(f) By incision to remove the pus and the use of antibiotics.

26 (a) Pitting oedema of the leg. Note the incision and suture above.

(b) Primary and secondary oedema.

(c) Primary oedema is caused by congenital absence or nearly so of the lymphatic vessels.

(d) The biopsy showed *the lymph glands replaced by cancer.*

27 (a) *Ligation of the patent ductus arteriosus.*

(b) Auscultation of a continuous murmur in the second left interspace and a loud second heart sound.

(c) By angiography.

(d) The recurrent laryngeal nerve, which curves round the ductus.

28 (a) A tiny orifice is present instead of the wide opening. This is *coarctation of the aorta.*

(b) By the absence of or markedly diminished femoral pulses.

(c) If it is mild there may be no symptoms for some time, but it could get worse on growth when cardiac failure may occur.

(d) The area of narrowing is excised and the aorta is reconstituted.

29 (a) *Osteosarcoma.*

(b) Males, aged 10–20 years.

(c) Yes, by the blood, especially to the lungs.

(d) Biopsy, radiotherapy and adjuvant chemotherapy.

(e) Yes, but many are associated with Paget's disease.

30 (a) *Enterolith obstruction.*

(b) A stone is formed in a duodenal or jejunal diverticulum.

(c) As the stone increases in size, it eventually blocks a narrow area, or it may pass onwards causing colicky attacks.

(d) This is possible but often there is little sign of this happening.

(e) Once diagnosed or suspected, an operation should be done to remove the stone because it may cause an obstruction in the lower ileum.

31 (a) A tumour in the right elbow.

(b) Secondary.

(c) In the bronchus, i.e. *bronchial carcinoma.*

(d) By radiotherapy and chemotherapy.

(e) Poor.

32 (a) *Sacrococcygeal teratoma.*

(b) The teratomas are congenital neoplasms of the basic cells of the embryo.

(c) In the gonads, the mediastinum, the retroperitoneal region and the coccygeal region.

(d) By excision, radiotherapy and chemotherapy.

33 (a) Biopsy established it as a *chordoma.*

(b) It is derived from the embryonic rests of the notochord.
(c) The base of the skull and the sacrococcygeal region.
(d) It grows very slowly and appears to be histologically benign.
(e) It is very difficult to excise because of its slowly invasive progress.

34 (a) The firm texture of the swelling suggested a sarcoma. It was present in the fat area rather than in the muscle.
(b) Biopsy showed the tumour to be a *liposarcoma.*
(c) It is well differentiated; myxoid, round cell, and pleomorphic (worse type).
(d) In the retroperitoneum and lower extremities.
(e) The 5- and 10-year survival rates are 50% and 5% respectively.

35 (a) *Sarcoma.*
(b) *Fibrosarcoma* is usually diagnosed, but it may be leiomyosarcoma.
(c) Wide local excision with adequate margins.
(d) The 5- and 10-year survival rates are 60% and 50% respectively.

36 (a) *Myosarcoma.*
(b) Rhabdomyosarcoma and leiomyosarcoma.
(c) Rhabdomyosarcoma is usually diagnosed as a soft-tissue sarcoma in children. Leiomyosarcoma resembles fibrosarcoma, and is usually found in the stomach, small intestine, and uterus.
(d) Rhabdomyosarcoma responds to radiotherapy and chemotherapy. Leiomyosarcoma is treated by excision, but recurrence is very likely.

37 (a) *Torsion of a mesenteric cyst and omentum.*
(b) The presence of an enlarging cyst can result in a torsion effect which includes the omentum.
(c) The drag effect may produce an intestinal obstruction.
(d) No, it is rare.
(e) Excision of the torsion area.

38 (a) *A subphrenic abscess on the right side.*
(b) Persistent fever after abdominal surgery or sepsis, with referred shoulder pain.
(c) Usually from complications of hepatobiliary or gastric surgery.
(d) A high leucocyte count and positive blood culture are suggestive. Chest X-ray, and a CT scan are definitive in diagnosis. An ultrasound and radio-nuclide scan will also help in difficult areas.
(e) Percutaneous catheterisation or, in some cases, open drainage.

39 (a) Sarcoma of the lower femur—Ewing's tumour. This is mostly seen in the second decade.
(b) Pain and swelling in the extremities, perhaps with fever at times.
(c) Destruction of metaphysis and diaphysis with periosteal new bone form-ation.
(d) Local and distal metastases, especially in the lung.
(e) Radiotherapy and chemotherapy, with possible wide excision of bone later.

40 (a) The arrow points to a *cancer of the ampulla of Vater.*
(b) The head of the pancreas.
(c) Intermittent jaundice, anaemia, and occult blood in the stools.
(d) A barium meal which shows a reversed figure three appearance, duodeno-scopy and histology.

41 (a) A clear fluid with a greenish tinge suggests a *pancreatic fistula.*
(b) Drainage of a pancreatic abscess near the tail of the pancreas.
(c) The fistula was dissected out, and the skin end of the fistula was inverted and sutured into the jejunum.

42 (a) *Cancer of the ureter*, from which secondaries passed to the liver and bone.
(b) Mostly transitional cell cancers.
(c) Haematuria.
(d) Urinalysis, IVP, cystoscopy and retrograde pyelography, chest X-ray, CT scan, and bone scan for metastases.
(e) At the lower end, just above the bladder orifice.

43 (a) *Hirschsprung's disease.*
(b) The absence of parasympathetic myenteric nerve cells in the colon and rectum.
(c) Males to females at 5:1.
(d) The clinical features are variable. Less meconium is passed, and there is marked constipation, abdominal distension and diarrhoea.
(e) A colostomy is done at the transition zone, and the presence of ganglion cells is noted.

44 (a) *Adenolymphoma.*
(b) It is slow growing, softer than tumours, and can have a cystic feel.
(c) Warthin's tumour.
(d) Tuberculous node or parotid tumour.
(e) Epithelial and lymphoid elements.

45 (a) Adenolymphoma, *mixed parotid tumour* or parotid carcinoma.
(b) It is firmer than adenolymphoma, slow growing, can be very large, and there is no pain.
(c) Irregular areas of epithelium, fibrous tissue and collagen.
(d) No. It may develop malignancy in months or years and may cause facial nerve paralysis.

46 (a) Swelling, inflammation, and pus exuding from the right *submandibular duct.*
(b) A plain X-ray, a sialogram, and culture of pus.
(c) Excision of the submandibular gland.
(d) Damage to the hypoglossal and lingual nerves.

47 (a) His *left facial nerve is damaged* by parotid cancer.
(b) Pain in the ear and the side of the face, and difficulty in controlling the mouth.
(c) He could not shave because of the pain and tenderness due to damage to the sensory nerve.
(d) Radical excision of the area of the tumour, with plastic surgery repair. Note, protection is needed for the left eye.

48 (a) *Scleroderma.*
(b) A collagen disorder that produces digital ischaemia caused by thickening of the intima and perivascular fibrosis.
(c) It involves mostly skin first and then the vasculature, affecting the fingers, hands and forearm.
(d) Coldness of the fingers and hands, progressive blanching of the fingers, later atrophy and ulceration, and finally loss of the fingers.
(e) Very little. Sympathectomy or steroids may help.

49 (a) A *sliding hiatus hernia* repair. Note the wide oesophageal opening.
(b) Reflux oesophagitis, dysphagia, sometimes anaemia. The features may be worse on lying down or bending.
(c) Paraoesophageal, and mixed hernias.
(d) Nissen fundoplication is the commonest one.
(e) Good results are present in up to 85–90% of cases.

50 (a) Complete blockage in the upper part of the oesophagus, i.e. *congenital oesophageal atresia.*
(b) The catheter is quickly arrested on its way down, confirming the atresia.
(c) (i) Atresia with tracheo-oesophageal fistula (TOF).
  (ii) Oesophageal atresia without TOF.
  (iii) TOF without atresia.
(d) The infant will exhibit coughing, salivation, and choking. Feeding makes the problem worse.
(e) Sump suction plus antibiotics is urgent. Gastrostomy plus division of the tracheo-oesophageal fistula is carried out. A later operation is an extrapleural thoracotomy and anastomosis of the two segments of the oesophagus.

51 (a) *Leiomyosarcoma.*
(b) The proximal and middle areas of the stomach, where bleeding may occur.
(c) It often grows to a large size and may be easily felt in the abdomen, especially if it grows outward into the abdominal cavity.
(d) Radical resection as it is resistant to radiotherapy. The 5-year survival rate is 50%.

52 (a) *Crohn's disease of the colon with skip lesions present.*
(b) Colonoscopy and biopsy plus a full assessment of the blood and the metabolic status.
(c) This form of colitis is rather uncommon. About 25% of patients have this type of disease alone.
(d) Toxic megacolon, which fortunately is rare.

53 (a) *Interno-external piles* and anal cushions.
(b) Bleeding on defaecation.
(c) *Per rectum* examination, proctoscopy, colonoscopy, and barium enema to exclude cancer.
(d) A high fibre diet, sclerotherapy, and, if necessary, haemorrhoidectomy with excision of the bulbous area.

54 (a) *Popliteal aneurysm.*
(b) Atheromatous disease of the artery.
(c) Thrombosis in the aneurysm or even rupture of the popliteal artery.
(d) Thrombus would occur from kinking of the knee, especially so with dehydration or polycythaemia. Rupture would occur from splitting of the atheroma and thinning of the arterial wall.
(e) Resection of the aneurysm and insertion of a graft.

55 (a) A *polyp on a long stalk.*
(b) Benign—usually so if on a long stalk.
(c) Spotting of blood in the faeces.
(d) Colonoscopy and biopsy.
(e) A double contrast enema.

56 (a) A *small carcinoma* on the left and a tiny polyp on the right.
(b) A change in the bowel habit or blood in the faeces.
(c) It is necessary to examine the patient carefully over time, using e.g. colonoscopy. This might be done perhaps 6-monthly for a year and then yearly for 3–4 years.

57 (a) *Anal fissure.*
(b) Severe pain on the passage of large faeces.
(c) Bleeding on defaecation or spotting of blood on clothes.
(d) Small size proctoscopy, and later sigmoidoscopy and colonoscopy.
(e) A soothing ointment, e.g. Anusol; the stretching of the anus; fissurectomy.

58 (a) *Leiomyosarcoma of the ileum.*
(b) Obstruction of the bowel and the presence of a mass in the abdomen.
(c) Total excision of the tumour mass and the involved bowel.
(d) Yes.

59 (a) Histology of the large mass excised showed it to be a *primary lymphosarcoma.*
(b) This tumour is classified as reticulosis.
(c) Abdominal pain, anorexia, loss of weight, and anaemia.
(d) Surgical staging, radiotherapy and chemotherapy.

60 (a) Extensive replacement of the liver by a tumour that does not look like carcinoma.
(b) *Carcinoid syndrome.*
(c) The appendix and the ileum, less so the jejunum.
(d) The level of 5-hydroxyacetic acid.
(e) All carcinoid deposits must be removed. Chemotherapy, fluorouracil, may help. Hepatic artery embolisation plus chemotherapy may palliate. If the abdomen is clear, a liver transplant may be considered.

61 (a) *Aneurysm of the thoracic aorta.*
(b) It depends on size of the aneurysm and the possible erosion of related bones. Coughing and haemoptysis may occur.
(c) By aortography and CT scan.
(d) Saccular and fusiform types.
(e) By control of hypertension. Saccular aneurysm can be excised or oversewn. Fusiform aneurysm requires replacement by a tube graft.

62 (a) On the left, a block in the right femoral artery; on the right, a bypass graft.
(b) Claudication of the calf muscles and pallor in the lower limb on exercise.
(c) Femoropopliteal bypass using the vein.
(d) Artificial grafts; angiodilatation; or coring out the blockage by pneumatic means.

63 (a) *Nissen repair* of a hiatus hernia. The fundus of the stomach is isolated by clipping the veins, and the fundus is passed behind the oesophagus and sutured to the other part of the stomach.
(b) Regurgitation of gastric contents giving rise to oesophagitis.
(c) When food is eaten it will fill up the fundus which, when full, will press on the oesophagus and thus prevent regurgitation.

64 (a) *Rupture of the spleen.*
(b) As a result of a blow in the lower left chest or upper abdomen, with possible fracture of ribs.
(c) Pallor, abdominal pain in the left hypochondrium but spreading through the abdomen and sometimes pain in the left shoulder (Kehr's sign), hypotension.
(d) Splenectomy in cases of severe damage. For less severe damage, the spleen can be incorporated in a mesh bag which may stop the bleeding.

65 (a) *Rupture of the liver,* gross damage is present.
(b) Control of the vessels in the hilum would allow sutures through a mesh or special plaques to prevent cutting of the liver by the sutures.
(c) Some packing behind the liver may stop venous bleeding.

66 (a) A ruptured *hydronephrotic kidney.*
(b) A fall, or a blow against a hard object. In this case, the patient fell while playing football.
(c) Severe pain in loin at first, then signs of blood loss and haematuria.
(d) Nephrectomy.

67 (a) *Extraperitoneal rupture of the bladder.*
(b) External injuries to a full bladder, often associated with a pelvic fracture.
(c) Suprapubic pain, muscle rigidity, and, usually, haematuria.
(d) In this case, the damage was minimal. The opening was sutured and a catheter was inserted. The prostate was enlarged and was dealt with later.

68 (a) *Rupture of the jejunum.*
(b) Blunt trauma in a road traffic accident.
(c) A pneumoperitoneum.
(d) As there is no devitalised area, a double layer of sutures using catgut and prolene is required.

69 (a) An almost complete block in the left lung and in most of the right lung.
(b) Pulmonary embolism.
(c) Thrombosis due to clots, seven days after parturition.
(d) Thrombectomy, via the pulmonary artery, incision and removal of clots.
(e) Despite thrombectomy the heart could not be resuscitated.

70 (a) Blood discharging from the nipple.
(b) A *duct papilloma.*
(c) By exerting pressure on different areas of the areola or the breast.
(d) Clear serous, milk, black or green, purulent.
(e) Retention cyst, lactation, chronic mastitis, and breast abscess, respectively.

71 (a) *Cystosarcoma phylloides.*
(b) Cystosarcoma phylloides is usually regarded as benign, but malignant changes may occur in 20% of cases.
(c) A huge fibroadenoma which changes into a fibrosarcoma.
(d) By a simple mastectomy, and histology.

72 (a) *Paget's disease of the nipple.*
(b) There is an eczematous condition of the areola and erosion of the nipple.
(c) No. A close up view shows there is raised tissue suggesting infiltration of the areola from a slowly growing underlying cancer.
(d) An underlying tumour mass.

73 (a) The triad of portal hypertension, oesophageal varices and splenomegaly.
(b) *Cirrhosis of the liver.*
(c) Haemorrhage; treated by tamponade of varices, sclerosing injections, and shunt operations.
(d) Portal hypertension and low albumin.
(e) Portocaval, splenorenal, or mesenteric caval bypasses to lower the pressure.

74 (a) *A tumour of the liver or the kidney.*
(b) IVP excluded a kidney lesion but the kidney was pushed down. Blood and plasma analyses were not helpful. A chest X-ray supported hepatomegaly.
(c) Laparotomy supported the presence of a huge tumour. The *hepatoblastoma*, involving 80% of the liver, was excised. The preserved specimen is shown.
(d) The child did very well for 2½ years following the operation, but then died with large metastases in the right lung.

75 (a) A mass in the right lobe of the liver, i.e. *hepatoma*.
(b) Upper abdominal pain, and enlarged liver.
(c) A liver scan, angiography, an alpha-fetoprotein (AFP) liver biopsy.
(d) Excision of the hepatoma if possible. If not, then ligation of the hepatic artery for palliation. Chemotherapy had been tried.

76 (a) *Cancer of the third part of the duodenum.*
(b) This is rare.
(c) Cancer of the ampulla of Vater.
(d) Leiomyosarcoma, and lymphomas.
(e) Resection of the cancer and duodeno-jejunostomy.

77 (a) *Cancer of the penis.*
(b) It is rare and appears at about 60–70 years of age.
(c) Rarely so.
(d) A squamous carcinoma.
(e) Excision of the tumour by partial or total penectomy, with possible radio-therapy of the lymph nodes.

78 (a) *Ischiorectal infection and abscess.*
(b) Damage to the anal crypts, and infection backwards into the pararectal space.
(c) *E. coli*, staphylococci, streptococcus, and, sometimes, anaerobes.
(d) Early incision because of the presence of the abscess. Antibiotics, and the cleansing of the cavity in a bidet.

79 (a) Either an inflammatory reaction or a torsion of the testis.
(b) No, it is rare in children.
(c) *Torsion of the testis.*
(d) Operation exposed a gangrenous left testicle and a twist in the spermatic cord. Orchidectomy was done.
(e) Make sure that the other testicle is satisfactory and is not likely to tort. The testis should be stabilised.

80 (a) *Hydatid cysts.*
(b) The tapeworm *Echinococcus granulosus* forms larval cysts.
(c) Dogs and foxes.
(d) Eosinophilia.
(e) In the liver (50%), in the lungs (20%) and in other organs.
(f) The Casoni test is 80% accurate. Serology tests may also be done.

81 (a) Pulmonary oedema.
(b) Overload of fluids and left heart failure.
(c) It increases the resistance in the pulmonary vasculature by pressure on the small bronchi.
(d) Increased risk of pulmonary infection.
(e) Diuretics, antibiotics and cardiac care.

82 (a) *A ureteric stone producing an obstruction.* Stones are usually composed of calcium phosphate, oxalate or urate.
(b) Pain in the loin, haematuria, and infection.
(c) An intravenous pyelogram, ultrasonography, and a CT scan.
(d) Conservative, ureterotomy, extracorporeal shockwave lithotripsy, neph-roscopy.

83 (a) *Gangrene due to cold injury.*
(b) Those exposed to the cold, especially elderly people; alcoholics; and psychiatric patients, as in this case.
(c) Warm the body but not the foot. Sympathectomy may help, as may vasodilators.
(d) Parts of the toes will separate, and surgery may be needed.

84 (a) Tapering of the arteries suggests *arteriosclerosis* in a diabetic.
(b) The tibioperoneal artery is very narrow, the peroneal artery is blocked, and the posterior tibial artery is very narrow.
(c) Diabetic neuropathy which may lead to gangrene.
(d) A burning sensation at night, loss of deep reflexes or vibration sense from below upwards, this loss of sensation leads to cracks, blisters, infection, and gangrene.

85 (a) *Thrombus in the popliteal artery* and a block in the end of artery. Narrowing of the anterior tibial origin and tibioperoneal stem.
(b) An atheroma plus a clot.
(c) Thrombectomy with the equipment to remove the atheroma, and reopening of the artery by special catheters.
(d) Those to exclude diabetes and coagulation defects.

86 (a) *A block in the left common iliac artery*.
(b) Claudication of the left leg.
(c) Yes. The right internal iliac artery is narrowed.
(d) An aorta–iliac bypass, or a femoro–femoral bypass.

87 (a) *A carotid body tumour*.
(b) A neoplasm of the chemoreceptors, i.e. a chemodactoma.
(c) Carotid angiography.
(d) At the carotid bifurcation.
(e) By surgical excision, except in the elderly where it may be left as it is slow growing.
(f) Damage to the hypoglossal nerve and damage to the arteries.

88 (a) *A porto-caval shunt*.
(b) To lower the pressure in the portal system.
(c) Portal vein obstruction, which can be caused by: severe alcoholism, biliary cirrhosis, Budd–Chiari syndrome, Bantes syndrome, or splenomegaly.
(d) Use of a Sengstaken–Blakemore tube with inflation of gastric and oesophageal balloons. Somatostatin and injection therapy into the oesophageal varices.

89 (a) *Radial artery aneurysm*.
(b) From trauma—either direct damage, or the use of catheters or needles for sampling blood. It is caused by cystic degeneration in rare cases.
(c) It really depends on the presence of an adequate ulnar artery. If it is inadequate, a graft could be used.

90 (a) *Excision of a pilonidal sinus*.
(b) Either as a chronic sinus or, less commonly, following an acute abscess.
(c) Usually those with dark hair, hirsute males predominantly.
(d) Excision of the tract allowing primary closure or healing by secondary intention. Baths, douches, and the use of a bidet will help.

91 (a) *A spigelian hernia*.
(b) This hernia passes through the linea semilunaris, and between the rectus sheath and the lateral abdominal muscles.
(c) Pain, possibly aggravated by sneezing or increased abdominal pressure.
(d) At rest tenderness may be noted over the hernial ring.
(e) Yes. Incarceration may occur.

92 (a) *Bilateral cervical ribs*.
(b) Thoracic outlet syndrome.
(c) The lower trunk of the brachial plexus. There may be intermittent compression of the subclavian and axillary arteries.
(d) Hairdressing, painting, building.

(e) Pain, paraesthesia, and numbness, due to the pressure on the lower part of the brachial plexus.

(f) By postural exercises. Also by resection of the cervical or first rib to relieve the pain.

93 (a) *Bilateral lymphoedema.*
(b) Congenital lymphoedema.
(c) Female.
(d) Lymphangitis and recurrent cellulitis.
(e) In the baby nothing, except perhaps elevation of the legs. In later years, intermittent compression may be used.

94 (a) *A fairly large gastric ulcer.*
(b) The black spot may have been where bleeding from an artery occurred.
(c) Partial gastrectomy.
(d) Biopsy to eliminate cancer.

95 (a) Two large *aneurysms* had developed *in the brachial artery*.
(b) That these were congenital aneurysms.
(c) Is there a familial relationship? None was found here.
(d) The aneurysmal artery was resected and a graft inserted.

96 (a) *A large incisional hernia.*
(b) A ladder pattern with an intestinal obstruction.
(c) Wound infection, respiratory problems, poor suture technique.
(d) Using monofilament nylon, the midline is closed by the near-and-far and far-and-near technique.

97 (a) *Omphalocele.*
(b) Prematurity and massive size of protrusion.
(c) Excision of the amniotic membrane and, if no anomalies are present, suture in layers.
(d) A fabric can be sutured over the defect and then covered with skin flaps.

98 (a) *A narrowing of the common bile duct just below the bifurcation.*
(b) The narrow area is smooth, suggesting a stricture, possibly inflammatory or due to cancer.
(c) Gradual jaundice, with gradual lightening of the stools. Distension of the gall bladder may be present.
(d) Transhepatic cholangiography or ERCP. Angiography will help to define the hilar anatomy.
(e) The tumour should be resected if at all possible and a hepaticojejunostomy performed; or a stent can be inserted through the liver to allow bile drainage.
(f) Very poor, a 10-year survival rate would be good.

99 (a) *Addison's disease or adrenocortical failure.*
(b) On the abdominal wall when pressure is put on the skin, and in the mouth. In the most severe cases, the pigmentation may be quite noticeable.
(c) Corticosteroids.
(d) Water excretion tests and low 17-ketosteroids.

100 (a) *Congenital diaphragmatic hernia.*
(b) As an extreme emergency in the newborn.
(c) Breathlessness, cyanosis, very poor respiration on the left side.
(d) An emergency upper abdominal incision; replace the gut and the left lobe of the liver, and suture the diaphragm. Not easy to do.
(e) The left lung has completely collapsed due to hypoplasia. It is not easy to inflate.
(f) The pulmonary hypoplasia.

101 (a) Precocious puberty i.e. *adrenogenital syndrome.*
(b) Excessive production of androgens, usually from adrenal hyperplasia. Tumours are rare.
(c) Ovarian or testicular tumour and adrenal carcinoma.
(d) By exclusion. Tumours are evident on CT or MRI scans.
(e) It differentiates adrenal hyperplasia from carcinoma by the fall of the secretion.

102 (a) Narrowing of the coeliac artery.
(b) Atheroma at the origin is the commonest cause. Sometimes a narrowing of the median arcuate ligament is present.
(c) Postprandial abdominal pain, sometimes called abdominal or visceral angina.
(d) Division of the arcuate ligament may be satisfactory, but most often a resetting of the major artery or an arterial bypass is performed.

103 (a) *A neuroblastoma of the adrenal.* The tumour is above the kidney next to a large blood clot.
(b) Usually in the first 5 years of life, in the retroperitoneal area and the adrenal.
(c) Yes, in about 70% of cases.
(d) A mass in the abdomen and secondaries in the liver.
(e) Resection. Radiotherapy and chemotherapy give very poor results.

104 (a) *A cortical adenoma (Conn's syndrome).*
(b) Hypertension due to retention of sodium, muscular weakness due to hypokalaemia, and alkalosis.
(c) From a low plasma renin level and a high urinary aldosterone level.
(d) Use of CT scan or MRI.

105 (a) *Cushing's syndrome.*
(b) Moon face, buffalo type obesity, striae, amenorrhoea in female, hypertension, glycosuria and osteoporosis.
(c) Hypersecretion of cortisol and corticosterone.
(d) Hypokalaemia, hypochloraemia and raised levels of 17-hydroxycorticosteroids.

106 (a) *A parathyroid adenoma.*
(b) Fatigue, polydipsia, polyuria, renal colic, bone pains.
(c) An increased parathormone secretion causing hypercalcaemia and a low phosphate level.
(d) Yes. It could show subperiosteal resorption of the phalanges, a lack of minerals in the bone, cystic changes, nephrocalcinosis, or lithiasis.
(e) Parathyroidectomy.

107 (a) *Thyrotoxicosis with exophthalmos.*
(b) The thyroid gland is firm and smooth; a thyroid thrill or bruit may be noted; tachycardia, nervousness, irritability, sweating, and loss of weight may be marked.
(c) With antithyroid drugs, radioiodine, and partial thyroidectomy.

108 (a) The thyroid.
(b) *Primary toxic goitre.*
(c) Thiouracil was given to render the patient euthyroid, later this was followed by Lugol's iodine and propylthiouracil, to decrease vascularity, for two weeks before surgery.
(d) Subtotal thyroidectomy.

109 (a) *A simple non-toxic goitre.*
(b) Physiological (puberty, pregnancy, menopause), endemic, or goitrogenic agents.

(c) Dysphagia or dyspnoea.
(d) The thyroid may be either smooth or nodular.
(e) Only if pressure symptoms are present, or there is a fear of cancer (aspiration cytology will clear this).

110 (a) *Nodular goitre.*
(b) Inadequate thyroxine production caused by living in iodine-poor areas.
(c) The duration of the condition, dysphagia, a change in the voice, the family history, a hard gland, previous radiation of the neck.
(d) Male. Children with previous radiation exposure are also at risk.

111 (a) *Colloid goitre.*
(b) It is a compensatory response to a lack of thyroxine.
(c) By aspiration cytology or open biopsy.
(d) Distension of veins.
(e) For relief of a large goitre, or fear of cancer.

112 (a) *Progressive or malignant exophthalmos.*
(b) Glucocorticoids in high doses.
(c) Despite ablation of the thyroid, the condition may progress to proptosis, deteriorating vision, corneal ulceration, papilloedema, and ophthalmoplegia and panophthalmos.
(d) A lateral tarsorrhaphy, retrobulbar irradiation, surgical decompression of the orbit.

113 (a) *Undifferentiated cancer of the thyroid.*
(b) It is more common to women of middle age.
(c) No, it is rapidly fatal.
(d) Pulmonary is the most common, cervical nodes also occur.
(e) Radiotherapy, but this has a rather poor effect.
(f) No.

114 (a) *Papillary adenocarcinoma of the thyroid.*
(b) *A total thyroidectomy.*
(c) It forms about 85% of the cancers of the thyroid.
(d) Often by the appearance of the glands themselves, even before the thyroid.
(e) It grows very slowly and may last for many years.

115 (a) A thyroid gland with *Hashimoto's disease.*
(b) An autoimmune disease with the presence of antithyroid antibodies.
(c) Use of thyroid hormone; if there are pressure symptoms, an operation may help.
(d) By needle biopsy.

116 (a) *Reidel's thyroiditis.*
(b) Cancer of the thyroid.
(c) By needle biopsy or open biopsy.
(d) Tracheal compression.
(e) Administration of thyroid hormones.

117 (a) Dry, grey, coarse hair; thinning of the eyebrows.
(b) *Myxoedema.*
(c) Low protein bound iodine, and elevated serum cholesterol.
(d) Hypothyroid patients may develop hypotension, hypothermia, and shock and hypoventilation which may produce CO_2 retention.
(e) Give thyroxine.

118 (a) The testis is normal, but there is a gelatinous area above it.
(b) *Carcinoma of the epididymis.*
(c) That not all swellings of the epididymis are inflammatory.

(d) Serum tumour markers are helpful, e.g. LDH, AFP, LcGB.
(e) By orchidectomy and removal of the spermatic chord. Follow up with radiotherapy and chemotherapy.

119 (a) *Teratoma of the testis.*
(b) It depends on the predominant type of cell; i.e. embryonal carcinoma, teratoma, and chorion carcinoma.
(c) Embryonal carcinoma; this recurs in 50% of cases.
(d) Cisplatin, vinblastine, and bleomycin in combination. This is said to have a 70% success rate.

120 (a) This is most likely to be *seminoma of the testis.*
(b) A firm painless mass in an enlarged testis, occurring in men aged below 40 years.
(c) An ultrasound scan showing retroperitoneal nodes.
(d) Human chorionic gonadotrophins, AFP (alpha-fetoprotein) and LDH (lactate dehydrogenase).
(e) Orchidectomy with high ligation of the cord, radiation therapy, chemotherapy.

121 (a) *Bilateral hydroceles.* The left side of the scrotum is larger than the right.
(b) In 50% of newborn boys; in 25% of adult males.
(c) Rarely, in about 2% of boys.
(d) Fluid is passing down from the peritoneal cavity into both the hydroceles.

122 (a) The scrotum is larger on the right side, redness is present, pain is less than in torsion, so this is likely to be *epididymitis.*
(b) Most likely via the urethra or prostate.
(c) Rapid onset of pain in the scrotum and scrotal enlargement.
(d) Relief of tenderness by elevating the scrotum.
(e) A technetium scan shows increased uptake in epididymitis, and decreased uptake in torsion.

123 (a) *A thickened epididymis* which shows no sign of inflammation.
(b) Tubercular epididymitis.
(c) Where there is pyuria without bacteriuria.
(d) Cystoscopy which will indicate the presence of tuberculous cystitis.

124 (a) *Bilateral hydronephrosis and hydroureter.*
(b) The urethral valves causing obstruction and renal failure.
(c) At the post-mortem examination.
(d) Urethroscopy, cystoscopy, and urethrography.

125 (a) *Polycystic kidney.*
(b) In infancy, as an enlarging mass.
(c) The lesion is ballottable, therefore likely to involve the kidney.
(d) IVP (intravenous pyelography).
(e) Haematuria and renal infection.
(f) A renal transplant.

126 (a) *A renal or splenic problem:* possibly a tumour or cyst.
(b) IVP and ultrasound scan.
(c) A large mass in the renal area with deformation of calyces. The other kidney was normal.
(d) *Diagnosis: a large renal cyst.* It was excised and the rest of the kidney was preserved.

127 (a) *Splenomegaly* which is not usually as gross as this in the western world.
(b) The circle marks the greatest depth of the spleen, the outer line marks the

anterior border.

(c) Cirrhosis, Hodgkin's lymphoma, sarcoma, chronic malaria, Felty's syndrome, glycogen storage disease.

(d) By investigations of the blood and marrow, fine needle biopsy, and finally laparotomy.

128 (a) *Lymphoedema of the left arm* plus cancer of the chest area.

(b) Usually seen years after a simple or radical mastectomy.

(c) Recurrence of the tumour over the mastectomy site and over the skin of the right breast.

(d) No. This is too extensive a problem and the patient may already have had radiotherapy. Palliation by hormonal treatment could be attempted.

129 (a) The trachea and lungs removed.

(b) Malignant tumour of the right lung.

(c) Secondary tumours are rare, but this may be from a neuroblastoma or liver tumour.

(d) Hepatoblastoma.

130 (a) *Adenocarcinoma of the kidney.*

(b) Haemorrhagic necrosis and degeneration of the tissues.

(c) Commonly the lungs, renal nodes, adrenal, opposite kidney, and long bones.

(d) Surgery—radiation is of little benefit. Vinblastin or interferon have both had some response, and there is hope for future agents.

131 (a) *Nephroblastoma (Wilms' tumour).* Usually occurs before age 4 years.

(b) A renal mass is felt which moves on respiration and is ballottable.

(c) IVP showed a destroyed kidney. Needle biopsy could make final diagnosis and ultrasound would help to guide the way.

(d) The tumour has embryonic tissues, muscle fibres, cartilage and bone.

132 (a) *Papillary tumour* in the pelvis, or *transitional cell cancer.*

(b) Haematuria.

(c) Radiolucent filling defect in the renal pelvis.

(d) Nephro-ureterectomy.

133 (a) Caliectasis of the left major calyx.

(b) *Tuberculosis of the calyx.*

(c) Culture of the urine may be positive, but sterile pyuria is not uncommon.

(d) Renal pain, haematuria, renal colic.

(e) Cystoscopy may see typical signs of tuberculous cystitis.

(f) Partial nephrectomy.

134 (a) *Renal tuberculosis.*

(b) The ureter and pelvis are dilated; the renal cortex is thinned and bulging due to scarring; hydronephrotic changes.

(c) Caseation.

(d) Because of complete renal failure.

135 (a) The patient had haematuria and was found to have a large mass in the loin.

(b) A tumour of the upper pole of the kidney—*hypernephroma.*

(c) IVP and a CT scan.

(d) MRI is useful for staging the disease; chest X-rays and a CT scan of the chest can confirm most common metastases.

136 (a) *Rupture of the urethra.*

(b) Extravasation of urine.

(c) Pelvic fractures cause membrane damage just below the prostate by direct injury.

d) Urethrography.
e) Major injuries may need suprapubic cystostomy. Lesser injuries may need bougienage.

37 (a) As the stricture was very tight, a suprapubic cystostomy was done.
b) The gradual use of urethral sounds.
c) Culture of the abscess. Histology of the ulcer if it did not clear up.
d) Venereal disease, e.g. gonorrhoea, which should be investigated.
e) Tuberculosis, schistosomiasis, cancer.
f) Urethral calibration, retrograde urethroscopy, and a voiding urethrogram.

38 (a) A dissecting aneurism of the aorta.
b) A splitting of the wall or the dissection of the aorta.
c) Usually distal to the aortic valve in Type A (60%), or near the left subclavian artery in Type B (20%). The remainder are in the descending thorax or the abdominal aorta.
d) A weakness of the aorta, cystic medial necrosis, plus hypertension.
e) Aortography, and in chronic dissection a CT scan.
f) Type A is urgent, whereas Type B can be dealt with in time.

39 (a) The testes are not in the scrotum at 6 years of age.
b) See if the testes could be milked down.
c) No.
d) The inguinal canals can be opened and any attachments can be freed up to let the testes come down into the normal place.
e) No. The results are not too good.

40 (a) The left side felt fuller, and like a 'bag of worms'.
b) *A left varicocele.*
c) From deficiency of the valves in the deep venous return to the testes.
d) The left, because the testicular vein flows at a right angle into the renal vein.
e) Probably do nothing. If pressed, sclerotherapy can be used.

41 (a) An attempt to replace the testis into the scrotum.
b) The right side of the scrotum is poorly developed. Also the testis is small.
c) About the 7th week of gestation.
d) The testis is exposed to trauma. Also the incidence of cancer in an *unescended testis* is up to 50 times higher than in normal situations.
e) At about the fifth year up to the seventh year.

42 (a) *Thoracotomy.* Large bullae in the lung.
b) Probably from emphysema, asthma or dyspnoea. It is not really known.
c) Pneumothorax.
d) By excision of the bullae. The minor effects may resolve but a chest tube may be needed to relieve pneumothorax.

43 (a) *Blue–black ischaemic area* and necrotic ulcer on the heel.
b) Ischaemia and pressure damage.
c) Assess coldness and sensation in the legs; see if the leg and foot pulses are present; assess diabetic status and neuropathy.
d) Arteriography to assess the flow.
e) By arterial surgery, lumbar sympathectomy, vasodilators, or dissolution of clots.

44 (a) The left ureter is compressed and the pelvis of the kidney is distended.
b) A mass pressing on the ureter.
c) Calcification identifies the mass as an *aneurysm.*
d) Because of pain in the left loin, renal colic was thought of.

(e) Although unusual, cases are known where an aneurysm has ruptured when an IVP was being done.

145 (a) A mass in the superior mediastinum.
(b) Neoplasm, aneurysm, goitre.
(c) Chest films, CT scan, scintiscan.
(d) *Goitre,* shown best by scintiscan.

146 (a) *A stab wound in the left axillary artery.*
(b) By dissection of the axilla and suture of the vessel. A patch angioplast was considered.
(c) Vein, radial, ulnar and median nerves, and the medial cutaneous nerve.
(d) Thrombosis of the artery or vein. Pulses should be recorded, and low dose heparin might be of help.

147 (a) *A strangulated incisional hernia.*
(b) Central abdominal colicky pain, with pain, tenderness and redness in the swelling.
(c) A strangulated loop of bowel was noted.
(d) Resection of the bowel and end-to-end anastomosis.
(e) By continuous prolene suture through all the fascial layers with the far-and-near technique.

148 (a) A solid tumour in the pleura, i.e. a *sarcoma.*
(b) Tumours in the lung may be squamous cell carcinomas, oat-cell carcinomas, adenocarcinomas, or undifferentiated cancer.
(c) They are rare and of various cell types. The most common are *lymphosarcomas.*
(d) Surgery plus radiotherapy.

149 (a) *Below knee amputation,* but followed by gangrene of the flap.
(b) The blood flow in the flaps was insufficient for healing.
(c) By accurate assessment of the blood flow and avoidance of infection.
(d) Thermography and/or radioactive isotopes.
(e) Re-amputation usually through or above the knee.

150 (a) *Thermography of an ischaemic limb.*
(b) The forefoot is black with no blood flow. The colours represent various blood flows, the red showing highest flow.
(c) On the medial side of the upper leg, blood flow was 24 ml, and on the lateral side, 12.6 ml; these are good blood flows.
(d) After successful amputation, the blood flow at below knee level was 30 ml showing that the red area was viable.

151 (a) *Dry gangrene of the big toe.*
(b) The area above is red from inflammation and is a good colour.
(c) Either leave the toe alone to fall off or, better, operate.
(d) If there is no smell or suggestion of pus, leave the toe alone until it is ripe for removal. Antibiotics should be given and the foot kept dry.

152 (a) A large pouch protruding from the pharynx.
(b) The elderly.
(c) Dysphagia, regurgitation after meals, intermittent swelling.
(d) X-ray with barium.
(e) The pouch arises above the cricopharyngeal muscle below the inferior constrictor muscle.

153 (a) An opening into the bowel, with a cuff of atheromatous material on the outside.
(b) *A fistula between the aortic aneurysm and the duodenum.*
(c) Haematemesis and blood per rectum.

d) Excision of the atheromatous fistula with suture of the bowel. The anurysm was removed and a graft inserted.

54 (a) *The superior mesenteric artery* is opened from the aorta, and there is a clot in the lumen.
b) Postprandial abdominal pain, i.e. visceral ischaemia. The pain starts about 15 minutes after eating.
c) It usually begins with solid food, later with soft food, and can be very severe.
d) By arteriography.
e) Endarterectomy will open the area, or a graft may be interposed.

55 (a) The saponification is present due to calcium soaps related to *acute pancreatitis.*
b) Severe acute abdominal pain in the epigastric area with nausea and vomiting.
c) Gallstone disease, and alcoholism. Also trauma, hypercalcaemia or hyperlipidaemia.
d) Serum amylase of over 1000 IU confirms the diagnosis, although in alcoholic cases urinary amylase may also be of help.

56 (a) *Annular pancreas round the duodenum.*
b) By plain X-ray which will show a 'double bubble' of large stomach and small first part of duodenum.
c) Gastroenterostomy or duodeno-jejunostomy.
d) Because there is a danger of pancreatitis or pancreatic fistula.

57 (a) Narrowing of the oesophagus—stricture.
b) Below the stricture is the fundus of the stomach with a hiatus hernia.
c) The stricture can be dilated, but the hiatus hernia must also be repaired. A thoracoabdominal repair would be preferable, allowing the stricture to be seen and a Belsey repair instituted.

58 (a) *Removal of caecal cancer.*
b) Obstruction, mass in right iliac fossa, tenderness, melaena.
c) Cancer of the colon is as common in females as cancer of the rectum is in males.
d) As the caecum is capacious, it may take some time before the diagnosis is made.

59 (a) *Carcinoma of the head of the pancreas.*
b) Jaundice, deep seated abdominal pain, and loss of weight.
c) CT scan, ERCP, possibly upper GI series and aspiration biopsy.
d) By Whipple's operation (pancreatectomy).
e) The 5-year survival rate is about 10%.

60 (a) *Cullen's sign,* seen in the perumbilical area.
b) It is related to a ruptured ectopic gestation.
c) The action of the pancreatic enzymes producing haemorrhagic necrosis.
d) A grey Turner's sign which is somewhat similar but seen mostly in the flank.

61 (a) An oesophagus with indentations due to oesophageal varices.
b) Bleeding with vomiting, collapse or melaena.
c) Portal hypertension.
d) A sengstaken tube can be used to control the varices by pressure.
e) Injection sclerotherapy and/or decompression of portal hypertension.

62 (a) An opaque area below the inguinal ligament.
b) Because of the barium.
c) Barium meal with part of the stomach in a *large femoral hernia.*

(d) Open the area of the femoral canal, replace the stomach and suture o patch the femoral canal.

(e) There is a fear of strangulation; or there may be a rupture by a blow, or a fall with the stomach in front of the femur.

163 (a) The upper lobe of the left lung is opaque and there is some effusion above the diaphragm. There is also mottling on the right side.

(b) *Respiratory distress syndrome* (RDS) with engorgement of the left uppe lobe.

(c) The patient has a multisystem illness, i.e. dyspnoea, tachycardia, and a low arterial oxygen tension despite a high oxygen concentration.

(d) Usually diffuse patchy shadows. The lung bases may be clear.

164 (a) *Rupture of the heart and transection of the aorta.*

(b) Immediate thoracotomy with maximum blood available.

(c) Haemorrhage from the heart, and difficulty from a blood clot round the transection.

(d) A balloon may be guided up the aorta to block the aortic hole and allow a suture or a clamp to the vessel.

165 (a) *A large aortic aneurysm.*

(b) An aortogram.

(c) Aneurysms can be complicated by rupture, pressure on the ureter giving renal pain or aorto-caval fistula.

(d) Insertion of a tubular graft or aorto-bifemoral or aorto-iliac graft, depend ing on the narrowing of the iliac arteries.

166 (a) *Diaphragmatic hernia.*

(b) Possibly through the parasternal hernia of Morgagni, the pleuro peritoneal area of Bochdalek, or by trauma.

(c) A hernia would be produced by severe blunt trauma or penetrating wounds.

(d) By a nasogastric tube, X-ray, and/or barium studies.

167 (a) A blow on the side of the face has produced a deviated *fractured nose*

(b) Pain, tenderness, swelling at the root of the nose. A sharp break may be felt over the bridge of the nose.

(c) The inside of the nose should be inspected for a septal haematoma which must be drained. Under anaesthetic the nose must be manipulated to it normal condition.

(d) This too must be pushed back into its normal position.

(e) Cerebrospinal fluid rhinorrhoea which would require antibiotics.

168 (a) A blow on left cheek has caused a *fracture of the zygoma.*

(b) No, because of the bruising and swelling. An X-ray would show it up.

(c) An incision is made above the zygoma and a lever is inserted to produce the proper alignment.

(d) The alignment may not be stable and may require wiring or support o fractured bone by packing the antrum.

169 (a) Bilateral maxillary fracture, known as '*dish face' injury.*

(b) Probably the face hitting a car widescreen.

(c) LeFort I, II and III, depending on the severity of the injury and the areas o bone separated.

(d) Reduction, immobilisation, splinting, either by internal or external methods.

170 (a) *Thoracic aneurysm.*

(b) *Syphilitic aneurysm.*

(c) The vertebra have been eroded over a long period of time.

(d) Much depends on the patient's general condition and age, the hazards of the operation, and the status of the problem.
(e) Excision and grafting.

171 (a) *Tetralogy of Fallot.*
(b) A large ventricular septal defect, pulmonary stenosis (the main problem), an over-riding aorta, and hypertrophy of the right ventricle.
(c) Yes; there are four operations that can be done, as above.
(d) Periods of hypoxia, cyanosis which is improved by squatting, and finger clubbing.
(e) Excellent. Over a 90% success rate.

172 (a) A narrowing in the oesophagus with the right film showing almost complete obstruction.
(b) Compression of the oesophagus by a vascular ring, due to anomalies of the aortic arch, causing dysphagia.
(c) *Dysphagia lusoria.*
(d) Inspiratory and expiratory wheeze, and stridor if the neck is flexed.
(e) Barium swallow shows an indentation at T_3 and T_4; oesophagoscopy and bronchoscopy may help. The anomalous aortic arch requires surgical correction.

173 (a) *Dry gangrene.*
(b) Thrombosis of the axillary artery.
(c) If a clot had broken off, impacting in the radial and ulnar arteries.
(d) Arteriography, and removal of the thrombus by a balloon catheter.
(e) Heparinisation during and after the operation.

174 (a) The development of a *false aneurysm* with a previous patch graft.
(b) A portion of the sutured vessel opened up and blood pulsated through.
(c) Infection; not present here—culture was negative.
(d) A further patch graft with secure arterial wall.
(e) A bypass procedure.

175 (a) *Temporal artery biopsy.*
(b) Because temporal arteritis was diagnosed.
(c) Severe headache, local tenderness, rarely redness.
(d) No. It may affect the carotids and their branches, thus causing local tenderness.
(e) Giant cell arteritis. Those aged over 60 years.
(f) Steroids.

176 (a) *Aortic stenosis.*
(b) It may be asymptomatic. If it is severe, angina and syncope or heart failure may be present.
(c) Prominent left ventricular impulses and narrow pulse pressure. A thrill may be felt along the left sternal border and a harsh systolic murmur may be heard there.
(d) Stenotic valve, supravalvular or subvalvular stenosis, and hypertrophic subaortic muscle.

177 (a) *An atrial septal defect.*
(b) Primum, secundum, and complete atrio-ventricular canal.
(c) Pulmonary systolic murmur, fixed splitting of second sound, and right ventricular heave.
(d) It is the most serious of these defects, with early heart failure, cardiomegaly and pansystolic murmur.

178 (a) *Mitral stenosis.*
(b) The narrowed valve produces increased back pressure in the lungs with

dyspnoea on effort, orthopnoea, and paroxysmal dyspnoea.
(c) An enlarged left atrium, prominent pulmonary vessels with pulmonary congestion, and an enlarged right atrium.
(d) The first apical heart sound is loud with an opening snap and a crescendo diastolic rumble.

179 (a) *Leiomyoma of the oesophagus.*
(b) With mild dysphagia.
(c) It is the commonest of the rare benign lesions of the oesophagus.
(d) Some by oesophagoscopy for other reasons, but large ones are shown by barium swallow as a smooth swelling.
(e) Thoracotomy. The oesophagus is opened, the mass is easily removed and the oesophagus is resutured.

180 (a) Cystic degeneration of the popliteal artery.
(b) Calf claudication and decrease of the peripheral pulses.
(c) Arteriography. This shows a localised area of popliteal stenosis with an hour-glass appearance. Cysts may be present.
(d) Arterial graft insertion.

181 (a) *Small bowel obstruction* was present from adhesions following previous operation.
(b) Central abdominal pain, vomiting, distension, and constipation.
(c) Early treatment with gastric and intestinal suction, fluid therapy, colloids, and finally operation.
(d) Vomiting with regurgitation into the lungs.

182 (a) Excision of an *aortic aneurysm and graft insertion.*
(b) Not now. The whole aneurysm is not resected.
(c) The sac is incised, a *tube graft* is inserted at the top and at the common iliac bifurcation.
(d) Provided the common iliacs are clear the whole operation is easier, with less dissection behind, and suture of the graft at the top end is also easier.
(e) An aorto-iliac or even an aorto-bifemoral graft may be used.

183 (a) *A block in the abdominal aorta.*
(b) Most likely an atheroma with narrowing and thrombosis.
(c) If it were purely thrombosis, a balloon catheter would pull the thrombus down to the femoral arteries.
(d) The atheroma, so an open operation is necessary.
(e) Palpation of femoral pulses would note a drop in pressures.

184 (a) A single mass is seen, with others hidden, and it looks solid.
(b) It looks like a caseating gland and therefore a *tuberculous disease.*
(c) The ileum; Crohn's disease.
(d) Tuberculous disease is not common is western countries. The symptoms are diarrhoea and abdominal pain.

185 (a) *A large subclavian aneurysm.*
(b) The type of aneurysm is due to poststenotic dilatation.
(c) Usually due to cervical rib or thoracic outlet syndrome, or syphilis.
(d) Thrombus formation with emboli to the upper limb with possible gangrene.
(e) Excision of the cervical rib, if present, or of the first rib, excision of the aneurysm, and graft.

186 (a) An operation for a *carotid endarterectomy.*
(b) For an atheromatous plaque with thrombi or marked narrowing.
(c) Mainly the common carotid and internal carotid. The external carotid is not quite so important.

(d) If there are severe problems, yes. If the problems are minor, then aspirin and dipyridamole may be satisfactory treatments.
(e) A carotid endarterectomy with or without a patch.

187 (a) *Fracture of anterior fossa.*
(b) Rhinorrhoea, a discoloration around the eyes after some hours.
(c) An X-ray of the skull, a CT scan, cerebral angiography, an MRI scan.
(d) The Glasgow Coma Score.
(e) Eye opening, motor response, verbal response, eye signs, lower brain stem examination, motor pattern, and transtentorial herniation. Each of these requires varying responses.

188 (a) A cystic lesion in neck, i.e. *cystic hygroma.*
(b) Dermoid cyst, branchial cysts, and thyroglossal cysts.
(c) Cystic hygromas and lymphangiomas transilluminate, but cervical cysts do not.
(d) Cysts are prone to infection.
(e) Cystic hygromas tend to disappear, especially if infection has taken place.

189 (a) *Meckel's diverticulum* attached to the umbilicus.
(b) Vitello intestinal duct.
(c) The intestine may be caught up in a loop, with intestinal obstruction.
(d) Inflammation, Meckel's diverticulitis, bleeding from the gastric mucosa in the duct affecting the ileum, perforation.

190 (a) *Buerger's disease (thromboangiitis obliterans).*
(b) Multiple segmental occlusions of the small arteries in the hands and feet.
(c) In Buerger's disease there is infiltration in all layers of the arteries by round cells.
(d) It occurs predominantly in young adult males who smoke heavily.
(e) Arteriography—shows the narrowing of the vessels from the knee downwards.
(f) Stop smoking, sympathectomy. The condition may lead on to amputation.

191 (a) *An enterolith in the small bowel.*
(b) From jejunal diverticulae, with accumulation of material in one.
(c) This stone may have arisen from a gallstone impacting in the diverticulum.
(d) Infection and inflammation, perforation or obstruction of the bowel.

192 (a) The tongue shows *leukoplakia and cancer.*
(b) Yes, leucoplakia is cancerous.
(c) Radiation therapy; with time, both the problems here cleared up.
(d) Roughly 50–90%, depending on the stage of the lesion.

193 (a) *A stomal or gastro-jejunal ulcer.*
(b) The appearance of gastric pain after time (months or years).
(c) Pain is usually severe and is felt more in the left hypochondrium.
(d) Gastroscopy and biopsy.
(e) To exclude cancer.

194 (a) *A secondary cancer from a previous carcinoma of the stomach.*
(b) It is sometimes called Sister Luke's cancer.
(c) Because she was the first to make clear the recognition.
(d) Palliative only, as a previous gastric cancer was operated on and secondaries are probably widespread.

195 (a) An epidural or extradural haematoma.
(b) An epidural haematoma follows a skull fracture and lacerations of meningeal vessel.
(c) Usually the posterior branch of the meningeal vessel.

(d) The dura is stripped off from the bone and further bleeding may produce a large extradural clot causing brain compression.
(e) Mortality may be very high (over 30%), if there is a delay in diagnosis.

196 (a) *Lymphoedema of the right leg* due to lymph node metastasis from previous cancer of the ovary.
(b) Cystadenocarcinoma, endometrial carcinoma, and undifferentiated adenocarcinoma.
(c) Metastatic cancer from the gastro-intestinal tract, pancreatic cancer and breast cancer.
(d) No. Quite often there is a delay in becoming aware of such tumours.
(e) By pelvic examination, ultrasound, or a CT scan.

197 (a) *An enlarged liver with multiple cysts.*
(b) Usually a single cyst in the liver but it can have large mass, or there are multiple cysts.
(c) With multiple liver cysts, polycystic renal disease may be present.
(d) Solitary cysts should be resected as they may be premalignant. In this case the cysts were deroofed.
(e) Care should be taken to make sure there are no parasitic cysts or cysts with bile inside.

198 (a) *Fracture of the left zygoma and the maxilla.*
(b) By plain X-rays.
(c) Apart from the black eyes, the left side of the face is swollen and blood was draining out of the left nostril.
(d) Diplopia and/or intraorbital anaesthesia may be present.
(e) Malar fractures may be levered into position or may require wiring or support by packing.

199 (a) *Carcinoma of bladder.*
(b) Males to females 2:1.
(c) The majority (over 90%) of these tumours are transitional cell cancers.
(d) Marked haematuria with clot retention, urinary frequency, and cystitis.
(e) By cystoscopy and biopsy.
(f) The treatment depends on the depth of the involvement of the bladder. Transurethral resection or laser therapy is used. Partial or total cystectomy, or the use of chemotherapy may be necessary.

200 (a) This was thought to be a cancer of the testis.
(b) A chronic epididymitis.
(c) On section of the scrotal contents the testis was normal and a tumour was almost surrounding the testis.
(d) Histology revealed a carcinoma of the epididymis.

Index

Numbers refer to the number shared by the illustration, question and answer.